101 WAYS TO FIGHT CANCER

'The Other C Word You Don't Want to Hear'

Contents

Introduction

Cancer. The mere mention of the word can send shivers down the spine, conjuring images of hospital rooms, chemotherapy sessions, and uncertain futures. It's often referred to as "the big C" — a disease that disrupts lives, challenges spirits, and tests the very limits of human endurance. For many, hearing a cancer diagnosis is akin to entering a battle without a clear roadmap or guaranteed victory. It's the other C word you don't want to hear, it marks the beginning of a journey defined by resilience, hope, and the relentless pursuit of life.

'Fighting Cancer' is a comprehensive guide designed to arm you with an array of strategies, treatments, and approaches to take on this formidable opponent. Whether you are a patient, a caregiver, or someone looking to support a loved one, this book aims to provide you with a beacon of light in what can often feel like a dark and overwhelming tunnel.

What is Cancer?

Cancer is not a single disease but a collection of related diseases that can affect virtually any part of the body. Its complexity and variability make it one of the most challenging medical conditions to understand and treat. To grasp the true nature of cancer, it's essential to delve deeper into its biology, causes, and the broader impact on individuals and society.

Cancer begins at the cellular level, where the normal regulatory mechanisms that control cell growth, division, and death malfunction. Under typical circumstances, cells grow and divide to form new cells as the body needs them. When cells grow old or become damaged, they die, and new cells take their place. Cancer disrupts this orderly process.

It starts with mutations in the DNA of cells. These mutations can activate oncogenes (genes that promote cell division) or deactivate tumour suppressor genes (genes that inhibit cell division). This results in uncontrolled cell proliferation.

The unchecked growth of cancer cells leads to the formation of a mass of tissue called a tumour. Tumours can be benign (non-cancerous) or malignant (cancerous). Malignant tumours can invade nearby tissues and spread to other parts of the body.

One of the hallmarks of cancer is its ability to metastasize. Cancer cells can break away from the original tumour, travel through the bloodstream or lymphatic system, and form new tumours in other organs or tissues. This spread complicates treatment and often signifies a more advanced stage of the disease.

The development of cancer is a multifactorial process, influenced by a combination of genetic, environmental, and lifestyle factors. Some individuals inherit genetic mutations that increase their risk of developing certain types of cancer. For example, mutations in the BRCA1 and BRCA2 genes significantly elevate the risk of breast and ovarian cancers. However, not all cancers are hereditary. Most genetic mutations associated with cancer are acquired rather than inherited.

The environment plays a significant role in cancer risk. Exposure to carcinogens, such as tobacco smoke, asbestos, and certain chemicals, can induce genetic mutations leading to cancer. Ultraviolet (UV) radiation from the sun and radon gas are also well-known environmental risk factors. Lifestyle choices can greatly influence cancer risk. Factors such as diet, physical activity, alcohol consumption, and exposure to infectious agents (e.g., human papillomavirus) can contribute to the likelihood of developing cancer. Obesity and a sedentary lifestyle have also been linked to increased cancer risk. The risk of developing cancer increases with age. Over time, the accumulation of genetic mutations and prolonged exposure to carcinogens can lead to the onset of cancer. This is why cancer is more commonly diagnosed in older adults.

Despite significant advancements in medical science, cancer remains a leading cause of death worldwide. According to the World Health Organisation (WHO), cancer accounted for nearly 10 million deaths in 2020, making it one of the most pressing health challenges globally. The burden of cancer is immense, affecting individuals, families, and healthcare systems.

The economic cost of cancer is substantial. The direct costs include medical expenses for diagnosis, treatment, and palliative care, while indirect costs involve lost productivity and income due to illness and premature death. The financial burden can be overwhelming for patients and their families, often leading to long-term economic hardship. Beyond the physical toll, cancer has profound social and emotional implications. A diagnosis can lead to anxiety, depression, and a sense of isolation. The journey through cancer treatment often involves significant lifestyle changes and can strain personal relationships. Support from family, friends, and healthcare professionals is crucial in helping patients cope with the emotional challenges of cancer. Cancer care places a significant demand on healthcare systems too. The need for specialised treatment facilities, trained medical personnel, and advanced diagnostic and therapeutic technologies requires substantial investment. Additionally, disparities in access to care between different regions and socioeconomic groups pose a significant challenge in achieving equitable cancer treatment and outcomes.

The fight against cancer is a global priority, driving extensive research and innovation. Scientists and medical professionals are dedicated to understanding the underlying mechanisms of cancer, developing new treatments, and improving existing ones. Cancer research is a dynamic and rapidly evolving field. Breakthroughs in molecular biology, genetics, and immunology have led to the development of targeted therapies and immunotherapies that offer more precise and effective treatment options. Researchers are also exploring the role of the tumour microenvironment, epigenetics, and metabolic pathways in cancer development and progression. One of the most promising approaches in modern oncology is personalised medicine. By analysing the genetic and molecular profile of a patient's tumour, clinicians can tailor treatments to target specific mutations and pathways. This approach aims to maximise treatment efficacy while minimising side effects.

Prevention and early detection are critical components of cancer control. Public health initiatives that promote healthy lifestyles, vaccination programs (e.g., HPV and hepatitis B vaccines), and regular screening tests (e.g., mammograms, and colonoscopies) can significantly reduce cancer incidence and improve outcomes.

The fight against cancer is a collaborative effort involving governments, research institutions, healthcare providers, non-profit organisations, and the private sector. International partnerships and initiatives, such as the WHO's Global Action Plan for the Prevention and Control of Noncommunicable Diseases, aim to reduce the global burden of cancer through coordinated efforts.

Cancer is a formidable adversary that affects millions of lives worldwide. Its complexity demands a comprehensive and multifaceted approach to prevention, diagnosis, treatment, and care. While significant progress has been made, the journey is far from over. Continued research, innovation, and collaboration are essential to overcome the challenges posed by cancer.

In "Fighting Cancer, The Other C Word You Don't Want to Hear," we explore 101 different ways to confront and combat this disease, from scientifically validated treatments to alternative and experimental methods. Traditional methods like surgery, chemotherapy, and radiation are cornerstones of cancer therapy, but they are not the only options. The fight against cancer can also include lifestyle changes, complementary therapies, cutting-edge technologies, and even unconventional approaches.

Navigating the Fight

Each person's battle with cancer is unique, influenced by the type of cancer, stage at diagnosis, overall health, and personal beliefs. This book does not advocate abandoning conventional treatments but rather seeks to complement and enhance traditional approaches with additional strategies that may improve outcomes and quality of life. The methods presented here range from mainstream medical treatments to holistic practices, dietary adjustments, psychological approaches, and even some unconventional ideas. The goal is to provide a well-rounded arsenal of options to consider in consultation with healthcare providers.

This book is not just about surviving cancer; it's about thriving in spite of it. It's about reclaiming control, making informed decisions, and fostering a mindset that embraces life with all its challenges and triumphs. Whether you are newly diagnosed, undergoing treatment, or supporting a loved one, may this book be a source of strength, inspiration, and actionable insights. Remember that you are not alone. The pages that follow are filled with practical advice and innovative ideas, a guide, a companion, and a testament to the resilience of the human spirit in the face of one of life's most daunting challenges.

Welcome to "Fighting Cancer, The Other C Word You Don't Want to Hear." May this book be your ally in the battle, providing you with 101 ways to fight back, stand strong, and live fully.

Scientific/Evidence-Based Treatments

1. Surgery: Removing Tumours Surgically

Surgery is one of the oldest and most common treatments for cancer. It involves the physical removal of tumours from the body and can play a pivotal role in cancer management. The primary goal of surgery is to excise as much of the cancerous tissue as possible while minimising damage to surrounding healthy tissue. There are various types of surgical procedures used in the treatment of cancer, each tailored to the specific needs and circumstances of the patient.

Types of Cancer Surgery

Curative Surgery: This type of surgery is performed when cancer is localised to one area of the body and is likely to be completely removed. Curative surgery aims to eradicate the cancer entirely and is often followed by other treatments such as chemotherapy or radiation to ensure any remaining cancer cells are destroyed.

Debulking Surgery: In cases where removing the entire tumour is not possible or safe, debulking surgery is performed to remove as much of the tumour as possible. This can help reduce symptoms and improve the effectiveness of other treatments like radiation or chemotherapy, as smaller tumours are easier to treat.

Palliative Surgery: When cancer is advanced and not curable, palliative surgery may be used to relieve symptoms and improve the quality of life. For example, surgery might be done to relieve a blockage in the intestines or to alleviate pain caused by a tumour pressing on nerves or bones.

Preventive (Prophylactic) Surgery: Some surgeries are performed to prevent cancer. For instance, individuals with a high risk of developing certain types of cancer, such as those with BRCA gene mutations, may choose to undergo preventive mastectomies (breast removal) or oophorectomies (ovary removal) to reduce their risk.

Diagnostic Surgery (Biopsy): Diagnostic surgery is used to obtain a tissue sample (biopsy) from a tumour or suspicious area. The sample is then analysed under a microscope to determine if it is cancerous and to identify the type and stage of cancer.

Staging Surgery: This surgery helps determine the extent of cancer spread. It can involve removing lymph nodes or other tissues to examine them for cancer cells. Staging is crucial for developing an appropriate treatment plan.

Reconstructive (Plastic) Surgery: After the removal of cancerous tissue, reconstructive surgery may be necessary to restore the appearance and function of affected areas. This is common in breast cancer patients who undergo mastectomy and opt for breast reconstruction.

Minimally Invasive Surgery: Advances in surgical techniques have led to the development of minimally invasive procedures, such as laparoscopic and robotic surgery. These techniques involve smaller incisions, which reduce recovery time, pain, and the risk of complications. They are used in various cancers, including colorectal, prostate, and gynaecologic cancers.

The surgical process typically involves several steps, each designed to ensure the best possible outcome for the patient. Before surgery, a thorough assessment is conducted to evaluate the patient's overall health, the extent of the cancer, and the best surgical approach. This may include imaging studies (CT, MRI, PET scans), blood tests, and consultations with various specialists. Depending on the type and extent of surgery, anaesthesia is administered to ensure the patient is comfortable and pain-free during the procedure. This can range from local anaesthetic (numbing a specific area) to general anaesthetic (putting the patient to sleep). During the operation, the surgeon makes incisions and removes the tumour along with some surrounding healthy tissue to ensure clear margins. The surgeon may also remove lymph nodes or other tissues to check for cancer spread.

Following surgery, patients undergo vigilant monitoring throughout their recovery period. This includes managing pain, attending to wound care, and observing for potential complications such as infection or bleeding. The duration of hospitalisation and recovery time varies based on the type of surgery performed and the patient's overall health.

Surgery typically serves as a pivotal part of an extensive cancer treatment strategy. It may be complemented by additional therapies such as chemotherapy, radiation therapy, hormone therapy, or targeted therapy aimed at eliminating any residual cancer cells and minimising the chances of cancer recurrence.

Patients receive close monitoring throughout the treatment regimen to manage any potential side effects and ensure the precise delivery of radiation. Follow-up appointments are scheduled to assess treatment response and address any long-term effects that may arise.

Risks and Benefits

Like any medical procedure, cancer surgery carries both risks and benefits:

Benefits:

Potential Cure: Surgery can be curative, especially if the cancer is detected early and is localised.

Symptom Relief: Removing or reducing the sise of tumours can alleviate symptoms and improve the quality of life.

Diagnosis and Staging: Surgery provides critical information about the type and extent of cancer, guiding further treatment.

Risks:

Complications: Surgery carries risks of complications, such as infection, bleeding, and adverse reactions to anaesthesia.

Recovery Time: Depending on the surgery's extent, recovery can be lengthy and may involve pain and discomfort.

Impact on Function and Appearance: Some surgeries, particularly those involving large or visible tumours, can affect the function and appearance of the affected area. Reconstructive surgery may be necessary.

Recent advancements in surgical techniques and technology have significantly improved the outcomes of cancer surgery. Innovations such as robotic-assisted surgery, which provides greater precision and control, and intraoperative imaging, which allows real-time visualisation of the surgical site, have enhanced the ability to remove tumours more effectively and with fewer side effects. Surgery remains a cornerstone of cancer treatment, offering the potential for cure, symptom relief, and valuable diagnostic information. As part of an integrated treatment plan, surgery can be combined with other therapies to increase the chances of success. The choice of surgery and the specific approach depend on various factors, including the type and stage of cancer, the patient's overall health, and the goals of treatment. By understanding the role of surgery in cancer care, patients and their families can make informed decisions and navigate the journey with greater confidence and clarity.

1. Chemotherapy: Using Drugs to Kill Cancer Cells

Chemotherapy is one of the most widely recognised treatments for cancer. It involves the use of powerful drugs to target and destroy rapidly dividing cancer cells.

Chemotherapy can be employed as a primary treatment, in combination with other treatments, or to alleviate symptoms in advanced cancer stages. Its application is broad, affecting a wide array of cancer types and stages.

Chemotherapy drugs work by interfering with the cell cycle, the process by which cells grow and divide. Cancer cells, which divide more rapidly than most normal cells, are particularly susceptible to these drugs. Chemotherapy can damage the DNA or disrupt critical cellular functions necessary for cell division and growth, leading to cancer cell death.

There are various classes of chemotherapy drugs, each with a different mechanism of action:

•   Alkylating Agents: These drugs damage the DNA of cancer cells, preventing them from reproducing. Examples include cyclophosphamide, ifosfamide, and cisplatin.

•   Antimetabolites: These mimic the normal substances within the cell, thereby interfering with DNA and RNA synthesis. Examples include methotrexate, 5-fluorouracil (5-FU), and gemcitabine.

•   Anti-Tumour Antibiotics: These are not like antibiotics used to treat infections but are drugs that alter the DNA inside cancer cells to prevent them from growing and multiplying. Examples include doxorubicin, bleomycin, and mitomycin.

•   Topoisomerase Inhibitors: These drugs interfere with enzymes called topoisomerases, which help separate the strands of DNA so they can be copied. Examples include irinotecan and etoposide.

- Mitotic Inhibitors: These drugs inhibit mitosis (cell division) and are derived from natural products. Examples include paclitaxel and vincristine.

Chemotherapy can be administered in various ways, depending on the type of cancer, its stage, and the specific drugs used:

Intravenous (IV): The most common method, where drugs are infused directly into a vein. This can be done through a peripheral vein or a central line, such as a port or catheter.

Oral: Chemotherapy drugs are formulated into pills or capsules that can be swallowed. This method is more convenient and can often be taken at home.

Injection: Drugs can be injected into a muscle (intramuscular) or under the skin (subcutaneous).

Intrathecal: This method involves injecting drugs directly into the cerebrospinal fluid to treat cancers affecting the brain and spinal cord.

Intra-arterial: Chemotherapy is delivered directly into the artery supplying the cancer.

Topical: For certain skin cancers, chemotherapy drugs can be applied directly to the skin.

Chemotherapy is often given in cycles, consisting of a treatment period followed by a rest period. This allows the body to recover from the side effects and healthy cells to repair themselves. The specific regimen depends on various factors, including the type of cancer, its stage, and the patient's overall health. Often, multiple drugs are used in combination to enhance efficacy. Each drug targets the cancer cells in different ways, reducing the likelihood of resistance and improving overall outcomes.

Neoadjuvant and Adjuvant Chemotherapy:

•   Neoadjuvant Chemotherapy: Given before surgery or radiation to shrink tumours, making them easier to remove or treat.

•   Adjuvant Chemotherapy: Given after surgery or radiation to destroy any remaining cancer cells and reduce the risk of recurrence.

Side Effects of Chemotherapy

While chemotherapy targets rapidly dividing cancer cells, it can also affect healthy cells that divide quickly, such as those in the bone marrow, digestive tract, and hair follicles. This can lead to a range of side effects:

Common Side Effects:

•   Fatigue: A pervasive sense of tiredness that does not improve with rest.

•   Nausea and Vomiting: These can often be managed with anti-nausea medications.

•   Hair Loss: Chemotherapy can affect hair follicles, leading to hair thinning or loss.

•   Anaemia: Reduced red blood cell count can cause fatigue and weakness.

•   Infection Risk: Lower white blood cell counts make patients more susceptible to infections.

•	Mouth Sores: Inflammation and ulceration of the mouth lining.

•	Diarrhoea or Constipation: Digestive disturbances are common.

•	Neuropathy: Numbness, tingling, or pain in the hands and feet due to nerve damage.

Advances in supportive care have greatly improved the management of chemotherapy side effects. Medications to prevent nausea, stimulate white blood cell production, and alleviate pain are commonly used. Nutritional support, physical therapy, and psychological counselling can also help patients cope with the physical and emotional challenges of chemotherapy.

The effectiveness of chemotherapy varies widely depending on the type and stage of cancer, as well as the patient's overall health. In some cancers, chemotherapy can achieve complete remission, while in others, it can significantly prolong life and improve its quality. Ongoing research continues to refine chemotherapy regimens, aiming to increase their effectiveness and reduce side effects.

Unlike traditional chemotherapy, which affects all rapidly dividing cells, targeted therapy focuses specifically on cancer cells with certain genetic mutations or abnormalities. This precision can reduce damage to healthy cells and improve treatment efficacy. Some chemotherapy regimens are now combined with immunotherapy, which enhances the immune system's ability to recognise and attack cancer cells. Researchers are also exploring the use of nanoparticles to deliver chemotherapy drugs directly to cancer cells, minimising exposure to healthy cells and reducing side effects.

Advances in genetic testing and molecular profiling have enabled more personalised chemotherapy regimens tailored to an individual's cancer type and genetic makeup, improving outcomes and minimising unnecessary treatments.

Chemotherapy remains a cornerstone of cancer treatment, offering hope and improved outcomes for millions of patients worldwide. Its ability to target and destroy cancer cells, either alone or in combination with other treatments, makes it a vital tool in the fight against cancer. Despite its challenges, advancements in supportive care and targeted therapies continue to enhance its effectiveness and manage its side effects, providing patients with a better quality of life during and after treatment. Chemotherapy is rarely used in isolation. It is often part of a broader, multidisciplinary approach to cancer treatment that may include surgery, radiation therapy, immunotherapy, and other modalities. This integrated approach is tailored to the individual patient's type and stage of cancer, overall health, and personal preferences, aiming to maximise treatment efficacy and improve survival rates.

Integration with Other Treatments:

• Chemoradiation: This involves combining chemotherapy with radiation therapy. Chemotherapy can sensitise cancer cells to radiation, making the radiation treatment more effective.

- Chemotherapy and Surgery: Chemotherapy can be used before surgery (neoadjuvant) to shrink tumours, making them easier to remove, or after surgery (adjuvant) to eliminate residual cancer cells.

- Chemotherapy and Immunotherapy: Combining these can enhance the body's immune response against cancer, providing a synergistic effect that boosts the effectiveness of treatment.

A critical aspect of chemotherapy is providing patient-centered care. This involves considering the patient's overall well-being, preferences, and lifestyle while planning and administering chemotherapy. Effective communication between healthcare providers and patients is essential to ensure that patients understand their treatment options, potential side effects, and the goals of therapy.

Medical Support: Regular monitoring and follow-up appointments to manage side effects and assess the response to treatment. Emotional Support: Access to counselling services, support groups, and mental health resources to help patients and their families cope with the emotional impact of cancer. Nutritional Support: Guidance from nutritionists to manage dietary needs and address side effects such as nausea or loss of appetite. Physical Support: Physical therapy and exercise programs to maintain strength and mobility during treatment.

Research and innovation continue to drive the evolution of chemotherapy, with promising advancements on the horizon. These include:

Biomarker-Driven Therapy: Identifying specific biomarkers that predict response to chemotherapy can help tailor treatments more precisely to the individual, potentially increasing efficacy and reducing unnecessary exposure to ineffective drugs.

Combination Therapies: Ongoing studies are exploring novel combinations of chemotherapy with other treatment modalities, such as targeted therapy, immunotherapy, and hormone therapy, to find synergistic effects that enhance overall treatment outcomes.

Drug Delivery Systems: Innovative drug delivery systems, such as liposomal formulations and biodegradable implants, are being developed to improve the targeting of chemotherapy drugs to cancer cells, thereby reducing systemic side effects.

Pharmacogenomics: The study of how genes affect a person's response to drugs is paving the way for more personalised chemotherapy regimens. Understanding genetic variations can help predict which patients are more likely to benefit from specific chemotherapy drugs and who might be at higher risk for severe side effects.

Chemotherapy has come a long way since its inception, evolving into a sophisticated and integral part of cancer treatment. Despite its challenges, it remains a powerful tool in the oncologist's arsenal, capable of saving lives and improving outcomes for countless patients. By continuing to refine chemotherapy approaches, integrating them with other treatments, and focusing on personalised patient care, the medical community strives to enhance the efficacy and tolerability of chemotherapy, bringing hope to those battling cancer.

3. Radiation Therapy: Using High-Energy Radiation to Kill or Shrink Tumours

Understanding Radiation Therapy

Radiation therapy is a cornerstone of cancer treatment, it works by delivering high doses of radiation to cancer cells. The radiation damages the DNA within these cells, preventing them from growing and dividing. Over time, the damaged cancer cells die and are naturally removed by the body.

There are several forms of radiation therapy, each tailored to the specific needs of the patient and the type of cancer being treated:

External Beam Radiation Therapy (EBRT): This is the most common form of radiation therapy. It involves directing high-energy beams (such as X-rays, gamma rays, or proton beams) at the tumour from outside the body. Techniques include:

•	3D Conformal Radiation Therapy (3D-CRT): Uses imaging to target the tumour precisely, minimising damage to surrounding healthy tissue.

•	Intensity-Modulated Radiation Therapy (IMRT): Modulates the intensity of the radiation beams, allowing for more precise targeting of the tumour and sparing of normal tissues.

•	Image-Guided Radiation Therapy (IGRT): Utilises imaging during treatment to ensure accurate delivery of radiation to the tumour.

•	Stereotactic Radiosurgery (SRS) and Stereotactic Body Radiotherapy (SBRT): Deliver very high doses of radiation to small, well-defined tumours, often in one or a few treatments. SRS is typically used for brain tumours, while SBRT is used for tumours in other parts of the body.

Internal Radiation Therapy (Brachytherapy): This method involves placing radioactive sources directly inside or near the tumour. It can deliver a high dose of radiation to the tumour while limiting exposure to surrounding healthy tissue. Brachytherapy is commonly used for cancers of the prostate, cervix, and breast.

Systemic Radiation Therapy: Involves taking radioactive substances orally or intravenously. These substances travel through the bloodstream to target cancer cells. Radioactive iodine (I-131) used in treating thyroid cancer is a common example.

Applications of Radiation Therapy

Curative Treatment: Radiation therapy can be used with the intent to cure the cancer, especially in early-stage or localised cancers. It may be the primary treatment or combined with surgery and/or chemotherapy.

Neoadjuvant Treatment: Radiation therapy given before surgery to shrink tumours, making them easier to remove.

Adjuvant Treatment: Radiation therapy administered after surgery to eliminate any remaining cancer cells and reduce the risk of recurrence.

Palliative Treatment: When a cure is not possible, radiation therapy can be used to relieve symptoms such as pain, bleeding, or obstruction caused by the tumour, improving the quality of life for patients with advanced cancer.

Total Body Irradiation (TBI): Used in preparation for bone marrow or stem cell transplants, TBI involves delivering radiation to the entire body to destroy cancer cells and suppress the immune system.

The Process of Radiation Therapy

The process begins with an initial consultation with a radiation oncologist, who evaluates the patient's medical history, cancer type, stage, and overall health. Subsequently, planning sessions (simulation) are conducted, utilising detailed imaging such as CT, MRI, and PET scans to precisely map the treatment area.

A multidisciplinary team comprising radiation oncologists, dosimetrists, and medical physicists then collaborates to create a tailored treatment plan. This plan outlines the specific type and dosage of radiation, the number of sessions required, and the precise targeting of the tumour.

During treatment sessions, the patient is positioned on a treatment table, and the radiation machine is aligned with the targeted area. The treatment itself is typically painless and lasts only a few minutes, though setup and positioning may require additional time.

Patients receive close monitoring throughout the treatment regimen to manage any potential side effects and ensure the precise delivery of radiation. Follow-up appointments are scheduled to assess treatment response and address any long-term effects that may arise.

Side Effects of Radiation Therapy

While radiation therapy targets cancer cells, it can also affect nearby healthy cells, leading to side effects. These vary depending on the treatment area, dose, and individual patient factors.

Common Side Effects:

•	Skin Changes: Redness, irritation, and sensitivity in the treated area.

•	Fatigue: A common side effect that can vary in intensity.

•	Hair Loss: Occurs in the treated area.

•	Digestive Issues: Nausea, vomiting, and diarrhoea if the abdomen or pelvis is treated.

•	Mouth and Throat Issues: Dry mouth, difficulty swallowing, and mouth sores if the head or neck area is treated.

•	Urinary and Bladder Changes: Frequency, urgency, or discomfort if the pelvis is treated.

Advances in radiation techniques have helped reduce side effects by sparing healthy tissue. Supportive care measures, such as medications, dietary adjustments, and skincare regimens, can also help manage side effects.

The field of radiation oncology is continually evolving, with research and technological advancements leading to more precise and effective treatments:

Proton Therapy: Uses protons instead of X-rays to treat cancer. Proton therapy delivers radiation more precisely to the tumour, sparing surrounding healthy tissue. It is particularly beneficial for treating tumours near critical structures, such as the brain and spinal cord.

Adaptive Radiation Therapy (ART): Involves modifying the treatment plan based on changes in the tumour size, shape, and position, as well as patient anatomy, during the treatment course. This approach enhances precision and effectiveness.

Flash Radiotherapy: An emerging technique that delivers ultra-high doses of radiation in a very short time. Early research suggests it may reduce side effects while effectively treating cancer.

Artificial Intelligence (AI) and Machine Learning: These technologies are being integrated into radiation therapy planning and delivery to improve precision, optimise treatment plans, and predict patient responses and side effects.

Radiation therapy is a critical component of cancer treatment, offering precise and effective methods to kill or shrink tumours while preserving healthy tissue. Its applications are vast, from curative to palliative treatments, and it continues to evolve with technological advancements. By understanding the principles, processes, and potential side effects of radiation therapy, patients and healthcare providers can work together to develop personalised treatment plans that maximise benefits and minimise risks. The ongoing innovation in this field promises to enhance

4. Immunotherapy: Boosting the Immune System to Fight Cancer

Immunotherapy represents a revolutionary approach in cancer treatment, harnessing the body's immune system to recognise and combat cancer cells. Unlike traditional treatments that directly target cancer cells, immunotherapy works by enhancing the natural defences of the immune system, offering a more targeted and potentially less toxic alternative.

The immune system is designed to detect and destroy abnormal cells, including cancer cells. However, cancer cells can develop mechanisms to evade immune detection. Immunotherapy helps the immune system to recognise and attack these cells more effectively. This can be achieved through various strategies, including enhancing the immune response, blocking inhibitory signals, or directly targeting cancer cells with immune components.

Types of Immunotherapies:

Checkpoint Inhibitors: These drugs block proteins that prevent the immune system from attacking cancer cells. By inhibiting these checkpoints, such as PD-1, PD-L1, and CTLA-4, checkpoint inhibitors unleash an immune response against cancer cells. Examples include pembrolizumab (Keytruda), nivolumab (Opdivo), and ipilimumab (Yervoy).

CAR T-Cell Therapy: Chimeric Antigen Receptor (CAR) T-cell therapy involves modifying a patient's T cells to express a receptor specific to cancer cells. These engineered T cells are then infused back into the patient, where they seek out and destroy cancer cells. This approach has shown remarkable success in certain blood cancers, such as leukaemia and lymphoma.

Monoclonal Antibodies: These laboratory-produced molecules can bind to specific targets on cancer cells. Some monoclonal antibodies mark cancer cells for destruction by the immune system, while others deliver toxic substances directly to cancer cells. Examples include rituximab (Rituxan) and trastuzumab (Herceptin).

Cancer Vaccines: Therapeutic cancer vaccines aim to stimulate the immune system to attack cancer cells. Unlike preventive vaccines, which protect against infections, therapeutic vaccines target existing cancer. An example is the Provenge (sipuleucel-T) vaccine for prostate cancer.

Immune System Modulators: These drugs enhance the overall immune response. Examples include cytokines like interleukins and interferons, which can boost the activity of immune cells.

Oncolytic Virus Therapy: This innovative approach uses genetically modified viruses to infect and kill cancer cells. The viruses can also stimulate an immune response against the cancer. An example is talimogene laherparepvec (T-VEC) for melanoma.

Immunotherapy has shown significant efficacy in treating advanced and metastatic cancers, including melanoma, lung cancer, kidney cancer, and certain types of lymphoma. It is often combined with other modalities like chemotherapy, radiation therapy, and targeted therapy to enhance effectiveness and overcome resistance. In some cases, immunotherapy is used as maintenance therapy to prevent cancer recurrence after initial treatment success which can be tailored to the individual patient's cancer profile, using biomarkers and genetic information to guide treatment choices.

Prior to commencing immunotherapy, patients undergo a comprehensive assessment to determine the suitability of the treatment. This evaluation includes examining the cancer type, stage, overall health status, and specific biomarkers that may indicate responsiveness to immunotherapy. Oncologists tailor a personalised treatment strategy based on the patient's unique cancer type and genetic markers. This plan details the specific type of immunotherapy prescribed, along with dosage and treatment timing.

Immunotherapy can be administered in several ways, including intravenously, orally, or through injections, depending on the specific treatment type. CAR T-cell therapy involves a more complex process where T cells are harvested from the patient, genetically modified, and then reintroduced into the patient's bloodstream. During treatment, patients are closely monitored to assess their response and manage potential side effects. Regular imaging studies and blood tests are conducted to evaluate the therapy's effectiveness and guide any necessary adjustments to the treatment regimen.

Side Effects of Immunotherapy

While immunotherapy can be highly effective, it can also cause side effects, often related to an overactive immune response. The side effects vary depending on the type of immunotherapy and the individual patient.

Common Side Effects:

•	Fatigue: A common side effect that can range from mild to severe.

•	Skin Reactions: Rashes, itching, and skin inflammation can occur, especially with checkpoint inhibitors.

•	Flu-Like Symptoms: Fever, chills, and muscle aches.

•	Digestive Issues: Diarrhoea, nausea, and vomiting.

•	Infusion Reactions: Reactions during or shortly after the infusion, including fever, chills, and difficulty breathing.

Immunotherapy can sometimes cause the immune system to attack healthy tissues, resulting in conditions such as colitis, hepatitis, pneumonitis, endocrinopathies, and skin disorders. Managing these immune-related adverse events (irAEs) often requires corticosteroids and other immunosuppressive medications. Early detection and management of side effects are crucial. Patients should promptly report any new symptoms to their healthcare team. Supportive care measures, including medications to control symptoms and adjustments to the treatment regimen, can help manage these side effects effectively.

The field of immunotherapy is rapidly evolving, with ongoing research focused on improving efficacy, reducing side effects, and expanding the range of cancers that can be treated:

Biomarker Identification: Identifying biomarkers that predict response to immunotherapy helps tailor treatments to individual patients, increasing the likelihood of success.

Combination Therapies: Combining immunotherapy with other treatments, such as targeted therapy, chemotherapy, and radiation, is showing promise in enhancing treatment effectiveness and overcoming resistance.

New Immunotherapeutic Agents: Research is ongoing to develop new immunotherapeutic agents and optimise existing ones. This includes exploring novel checkpoint inhibitors, CAR T-cell therapies, and oncolytic viruses.

Personalised Immunotherapy: Advances in genomics and molecular biology are paving the way for highly personalised immunotherapy approaches, where treatments are tailored to the specific genetic and molecular characteristics of a patient's cancer.

Overcoming Resistance: Understanding and overcoming resistance to immunotherapy is a major focus. Strategies include targeting additional immune checkpoints, modifying the tumour microenvironment, and combining immunotherapy with other treatments.

Immunotherapy represents a paradigm shift in cancer treatment, offering new hope to patients with various types of cancer. By harnessing the power of the immune system, immunotherapy can provide targeted and effective treatment with the potential for long-lasting responses. As research and innovation continue to advance this field, immunotherapy is poised to play an increasingly central role in the fight against cancer, offering improved outcomes and new possibilities for patients worldwide. Through a combination of scientific rigor, personalised care, and innovative treatments, the potential of immunotherapy to transform cancer care is immense and continues to inspire hope and progress in oncology.

5. Targeted Therapy: Drugs That Target Specific Cancer Cell Mechanisms

Targeted therapy works by interfering with specific molecules involved in the growth, progression, and spread of cancer. These molecules, often referred to as "molecular targets," can include proteins, enzymes, or genes that are mutated or overexpressed in cancer cells. Unlike traditional chemotherapy, which affects all rapidly dividing cells, targeted therapy aims to interfere with specific proteins, genes, or cellular pathways that are unique to cancer cells. This precision reduces damage to normal cells and can improve treatment efficacy.

By blocking these targets, targeted therapies can:

• Inhibit cancer cell growth and division.

• Induce cancer cell death.

• Prevent cancer cells from spreading to other parts of the body.

• Enhance the immune system's ability to recognise and attack cancer cells.

Types of Targeted Therapy:

Tyrosine Kinase Inhibitors (TKIs): These drugs block the action of tyrosine kinases, enzymes that play a crucial role in cell signalling pathways involved in cancer cell growth and survival. Examples include:

•   Imatinib (Gleevec): Used to treat chronic myeloid leukaemia (CML) and gastrointestinal stromal tumours (GISTs) by targeting the BCR-ABL fusion protein.

•   Erlotinib (Tarceva) and Gefitinib (Iressa): Target the epidermal growth factor receptor (EGFR) in non-small cell lung cancer (NSCLC).

Monoclonal Antibodies: These are laboratory-produced molecules that can bind specifically to target antigens on cancer cells. Some monoclonal antibodies deliver toxic substances directly to cancer cells, while others block growth signals or recruit immune cells to attack cancer cells. Examples include:

•   Trastusumab (Herceptin): Targets the HER2/neu receptor in breast and gastric cancers.

•   Rituximab (Rituxan): Targets the CD20 protein on B cells in certain types of non-Hodgkin lymphoma and chronic lymphocytic leukaemia (CLL).

Angiogenesis Inhibitors: These drugs inhibit the growth of new blood vessels (angiogenesis) that tumours need to grow and spread. By cutting off the blood supply, they can starve tumours of nutrients and oxygen. Examples include:

•   Bevacizumab (Avastin): Targets vascular endothelial growth factor (VEGF) to inhibit angiogenesis in various cancers, including colorectal, lung, and kidney cancers.

Proteasome Inhibitors: These drugs block the action of proteasomes, which are protein complexes involved in degrading unneeded or damaged proteins. By inhibiting proteasomes, these drugs can induce cancer cell death. Examples include:

•   Bortezomib (Velcade): Used to treat multiple myeloma and mantle cell lymphoma.

PARP Inhibitors: These drugs inhibit poly (ADP-ribose) polymerase (PARP), an enzyme involved in DNA repair. By blocking PARP, these drugs make it difficult for cancer cells to repair damaged DNA, leading to cell death. Examples include:

•   Olaparib (Lynparza) and Niraparib (Zejula): Used in ovarian and breast cancers with BRCA mutations.

Targeted therapies are highly effective in cancers with specific genetic mutations or molecular characteristics. They are often used in cancers such as breast cancer (HER2-positive), lung cancer (EGFR mutations or ALK rearrangements), and chronic myeloid leukaemia (BCR-ABL fusion gene). This therapy can be used alone or in combination with other treatments like chemotherapy, radiation therapy, and immunotherapy to enhance effectiveness and overcome resistance. In some cases, targeted therapy is used as maintenance therapy to prevent cancer recurrence after initial successful treatment.

Targeted therapy is a key component of personalised medicine, where treatment is tailored to the genetic profile of the patient's cancer. This approach increases the likelihood of treatment success and reduces unnecessary side effects. Before starting targeted therapy, patients typically undergo genetic and molecular testing to identify specific mutations or markers in their cancer cells.

Oncologists would develop a personalised treatment plan based on the genetic and molecular profile of the patient's cancer. This plan outlines the specific targeted therapy, dosage, and treatment schedule. Targeted therapies can be administered orally (as pills) or intravenously (through infusions). The method of administration depends on the specific drug and the patient's condition. Patients are closely monitored for response to treatment and potential side effects. Regular imaging and blood tests help assess the effectiveness of the therapy and guide adjustments to the treatment plan.

Side Effects of Targeted Therapy

While targeted therapy is generally more selective and less toxic than traditional chemotherapy, it can still cause side effects. These vary depending on the specific drug and the individual patient.

Common Side Effects:

•	Skin Problems: Rash, dry skin, and itching are common, especially with EGFR inhibitors.

•	Diarrhoea: Frequent with certain targeted therapies.

•	Liver Problems: Elevated liver enzymes indicating liver stress or damage.

•	High Blood Pressure: Common with angiogenesis inhibitors.

- Fatigue: A common side effect that can range from mild to severe.

The field of targeted therapy is rapidly advancing, with ongoing research aimed at discovering new targets, developing more effective drugs, and overcoming resistance. Advances in genomic technologies like next-generation sequencing (NGS) allow for comprehensive tumour profiling, identifying multiple potential targets for therapy. Researchers are also exploring the benefits of combining targeted therapies with immunotherapy and chemotherapy to improve treatment efficacy and combat resistance. Continuous identification of new molecular targets and advancements in targeted therapy development are expanding treatment options for patients.

A significant focus is on understanding how cancer cells develop resistance to targeted therapies. Efforts are directed at developing drugs that target alternative pathways and using combinations of multiple targeted therapies. The integration of targeted therapy within precision oncology approaches aims to personalise treatments according to each patient's cancer genetic and molecular profile, enhancing outcomes and minimising unnecessary treatments.

Targeted therapy represents a significant advancement in cancer treatment, offering a more precise and less toxic alternative to traditional therapies. By focusing on specific molecular mechanisms critical to cancer cell survival and growth, targeted therapies can effectively treat various cancers with specific genetic alterations. As research and technology continue to advance, the potential of targeted therapy to improve patient outcomes and transform cancer care is immense, providing new hope and possibilities in the fight against cancer. Through personalised approaches and innovative treatments, targeted therapy continues to evolve, offering a brighter future for cancer patients worldwide.

6. Hormone Therapy: Blocking Hormones That Fuel Certain Cancers

Hormone therapy, also known as endocrine therapy, is a treatment approach that targets cancers driven by hormones. Certain cancers, such as breast and prostate cancers, depend on hormones like oestrogen, (also known as estrogen), progesterone, and testosterone for their growth and survival. Hormone therapy works by blocking the body's natural hormones or lowering their levels to slow down or stop the growth of hormone-sensitive tumours. This treatment can be highly effective and is often used in combination with other therapies to enhance its efficacy.

Hormone therapy disrupts the hormonal signals that cancer cells rely on for growth. This can be achieved through various strategies:

•	Blocking Hormone Receptors: Some drugs bind to hormone receptors on cancer cells, preventing natural hormones from attaching and stimulating cancer growth.

•	Lowering Hormone Levels: Other drugs or surgical procedures can reduce the production of hormones in the body.

•	Inhibiting Hormone Production: Certain drugs can block the enzymes involved in hormone synthesis, reducing hormone levels.

Types of Hormone Therapy:

Selective Oestrogen Receptor Modulators (SERMs): These drugs block oestrogen receptors on breast cancer cells, preventing oestrogen from binding and promoting tumour growth. Examples include:

•	Tamoxifen: Commonly used for both premenopausal and postmenopausal women with hormone receptor-positive breast cancer.

Aromatase Inhibitors: These drugs reduce oestrogen levels by inhibiting the enzyme aromatase, which converts androgens into oestrogen in postmenopausal women. Examples include:

•	Anastrozole (Arimidex), Letrozole (Femara), and Exemestane (Aromasin): Used primarily in postmenopausal women with hormone receptor-positive breast cancer.

Oestrogen Receptor Antagonists: These drugs block and degrade oestrogen receptors, reducing the effects of oestrogen on breast cancer cells. Examples include:

•	Fulvestrant (Faslodex): Used for postmenopausal women with hormone receptor-positive metastatic breast cancer.

Androgen Deprivation Therapy (ADT): This approach reduces androgen levels or blocks androgen receptors to treat prostate cancer. Strategies include:

•	Luteinising Hormone-Releasing Hormone (LHRH) Agonists and Antagonists: Drugs like leuprolide (Lupron) and degarelix (Firmagon) lower testosterone levels by acting on the pituitary gland.

• Anti-Androgens: Drugs like bicalutamide (Casodex) and enzalutamide (Xtandi) block androgen receptors on prostate cancer cells.

Progestins: Synthetic progesterone-like drugs used in the treatment of certain cancers, such as endometrial cancer, that respond to progesterone.

Applications of Hormone Therapy

Breast Cancer: Hormone therapy is a standard treatment for hormone receptor-positive breast cancer. It can be used in various stages:

• Adjuvant Therapy: Administered after surgery to reduce the risk of recurrence.

• Neoadjuvant Therapy: Given before surgery to shrink tumours.

• Metastatic Breast Cancer: Used to control disease spread and alleviate symptoms.

Prostate Cancer: Hormone therapy is commonly used for advanced or metastatic prostate cancer. It can also be used:

• As Primary Therapy: For men who are not candidates for surgery or radiation.

• Adjuvant Therapy: Alongside radiation therapy to improve outcomes.

• Intermittent Therapy: To manage hormone-sensitive prostate cancer with periods of treatment and breaks.

(Hormone therapy may be used in certain cases of endometrial or ovarian cancers that respond to hormonal changes).

Before initiating hormone therapy, patients undergo testing to ascertain whether their cancer cells are responsive to hormones. This involves examining hormone receptors (oestrogen, progesterone, androgen) present on the cancer cells. Based on the cancer type, hormone receptor status, and individual patient characteristics, oncologists design a personalised treatment regimen. This plan details the specific hormone therapy prescribed, including dosage and administration schedule, which may involve pills, injections, or implants depending on the drug and patient's needs.

Patients receive close monitoring to evaluate treatment response and manage potential side effects. Regular follow-up appointments and tests are conducted to assess therapy effectiveness and make necessary adjustments to the treatment strategy.

While hormone therapy is generally well-tolerated, it can cause side effects due to changes in hormone levels. These vary depending on the specific drug and the individual patient.

Common Side Effects:

•	Hot Flashes: Common with treatments that lower oestrogen or testosterone levels.

•	Bone Loss: Hormone therapy can lead to decreased bone density, increasing the risk of fractures.

•   Joint and Muscle Pain: Often experienced with aromatase inhibitors.

•   Weight Gain: Can occur with certain hormone therapies.

•   Mood Changes: Including depression and anxiety.

•   Sexual Dysfunction: Reduced libido and erectile dysfunction in men, vaginal dryness, and decreased sexual desire in women.

The field of hormone therapy is continually evolving, with ongoing research focused on improving efficacy, reducing side effects, and expanding the range of cancers that can be treated:

The development of next-generation hormone therapies aims to enhance effectiveness and reduce side effects. These new therapies include selective oestrogen receptor degraders (SERDs) and novel anti-androgens. Research is also exploring the benefits of combining hormone therapy with targeted therapy and immunotherapy to improve outcomes and overcome resistance.

Advances in genomics and molecular biology are paving the way for personalised hormone therapy, where treatments are tailored to the specific genetic and molecular characteristics of a patient's cancer. Identifying and overcoming resistance to hormone therapy is a major focus, with strategies including the development of drugs targeting alternative pathways and the combination of multiple hormone therapies.

Hormone therapy is a vital component of cancer treatment, offering an effective way to slow down or stop the growth of hormone-sensitive tumours. By blocking the hormones that fuel certain cancers, this therapy can improve patient outcomes and quality of life. As research and technology continue to advance, the potential of hormone therapy to enhance cancer care is immense, providing new hope and possibilities in the fight against cancer

7. Stem Cell Transplant: Replacing Damaged Bone Marrow with Healthy Cells

Stem cell transplant, also known as hematopoietic stem cell transplant (HSCT), is a procedure used to replace damaged or diseased bone marrow with healthy stem cells. Stem cells are immature cells that can develop into different types of blood cells, including red blood cells, white blood cells, and platelets. This treatment is primarily used to treat cancers that affect the blood and immune system, such as leukaemia, lymphoma, and multiple myeloma.

Stem cells for transplantation can either come from the patient's own bone marrow (autologous transplant) or from a donor (allogeneic transplant). In autologous transplants, the patient's own stem cells are harvested prior to treatment. For allogeneic transplants, stem cells are obtained from a compatible donor, typically a family member or unrelated donor. Before the transplant procedure, patients undergo intensive chemotherapy and/or radiation therapy to eradicate cancer cells and suppress the immune system. This aggressive treatment also eliminates any remaining bone marrow. Healthy stem cells are then infused into the patient's bloodstream via a central venous catheter. These cells migrate to the bone marrow, where they initiate the production of new blood cells. This process, called engraftment, typically takes several weeks.

Throughout the recovery period, patients are closely monitored for signs of engraftment, infection, and other potential complications. Supportive care, including antibiotics, blood transfusions, and medications to prevent graft-versus-host disease (GVHD) in allogeneic transplants, is administered as necessary.

Types of Stem Cell Transplants:

Autologous Stem Cell Transplant: In this procedure, the patient's own stem cells are collected before high-dose chemotherapy or radiation therapy. After treatment, the harvested stem cells are returned to the patient to rebuild the bone marrow and restore blood cell production.

Allogeneic Stem Cell Transplant: In allogeneic transplants, stem cells are obtained from a compatible donor, such as a sibling or unrelated volunteer with closely matched human leukocyte antigen (HLA) markers. This type of transplant offers the potential for an immune response against cancer cells (graft-versus-tumour effect) but also carries a risk of GVHD, where donor immune cells attack the recipient's tissues.

Mini Transplant (Reduced-Intensity Conditioning): Also known as a non-myeloablative transplant, this approach uses lower doses of chemotherapy and radiation therapy before transplant. It allows older patients or those with other health issues to undergo stem cell transplant with reduced risk of complications.

Applications of Stem Cell Transplant

Leukaemia: Stem cell transplant is commonly used to treat acute and chronic leukaemia's that have not responded to standard treatments. It can be curative in some cases by replacing cancerous cells with healthy stem cells.

Lymphoma: Certain types of lymphomas, such as Hodgkin lymphoma and high-risk non-Hodgkin lymphomas, may be treated with stem cell transplant after initial chemotherapy or in cases of relapse.

Multiple Myeloma: Stem cell transplant may be recommended for younger patients with multiple myeloma to achieve remission or prolong survival.

Other Blood and Immune System Disorders: Stem cell transplant can also be used to treat other conditions affecting the blood and immune system, including aplastic anaemia and certain inherited disorders.

Patients undergo a thorough assessment to evaluate their overall health, disease status, and suitability for transplantation. This includes examinations to determine the extent of cancer, organ function, and compatibility with potential donors. In autologous transplants, stem cells are collected from the patient's bone marrow or peripheral blood using a procedure called apheresis. For allogeneic transplants, stem cells are sourced from a matched donor through bone marrow harvest or peripheral blood collection.

Following collection, patients undergo intensive chemotherapy and/or radiation therapy to eradicate cancer cells and prepare the bone marrow for transplant. The intensity of this conditioning regimen varies based on cancer type, stage, and the patient's health status. Stem cells are then infused into the patient's bloodstream via a central venous catheter, akin to receiving a blood transfusion, typically taking several hours. Patients are closely monitored in the hospital during the initial recovery phase, which may span several weeks to months. Regular blood tests assess engraftment and immune system recovery.

Supportive care, including antibiotics, antiviral medications, and growth factors, is administered to prevent infections and manage treatment side effects. After hospital discharge, patients receive ongoing monitoring for potential complications such as infections, GVHD (in allogeneic transplants), and long-term effects of treatment.

Advancements in Stem Cell Transplant

The field of stem cell transplant continues to evolve with ongoing research focused on improving outcomes, reducing complications, and expanding the use of transplant in various cancers and diseases:

Reduced-Intensity Conditioning: Advances in conditioning regimens allow for safer transplant options, particularly for older patients or those with pre-existing health conditions.

Cord Blood Transplant: Umbilical cord blood, which contains stem cells, can be used as an alternative source for transplant, especially when a suitable adult donor is not available.

Haploidentical Transplant: Transplants from partially matched donors (haploidentical) are being increasingly used, expanding the donor pool and improving access to transplant for more patients.

CAR T-Cell Therapy: This innovative approach involves modifying a patient's T cells to recognise and attack cancer cells. CAR T-cell therapy is showing promise in treating certain types of leukaemia and lymphoma, potentially reducing the need for stem cell transplant in some cases.

Stem cell transplant is a powerful treatment option for cancers affecting the blood and immune system, offering the potential for cure or long-term remission. By replacing damaged bone marrow with healthy stem cells, this procedure restores the body's ability to produce healthy blood cells and fight cancer effectively.

8. Precision Medicine: Personalised Treatment Based on Genetic Profiles

Precision medicine, also known as personalised medicine, is an innovative approach to medical treatment that takes into account individual variability in genes, environment, and lifestyle for each person. In oncology, precision medicine aims to tailor treatment strategies based on the unique genetic makeup of a patient's cancer cells. By identifying specific genetic alterations or biomarkers driving the growth and spread of cancer, oncologists can select therapies that are more likely to be effective and less toxic compared to traditional treatments.

This allows oncologists to do genetic testing which helps identify specific mutations, gene amplifications, deletions, or rearrangements that contribute to cancer development and progression. Based on the genetic profile of the tumour, oncologists can select targeted therapies or other personalised treatment approaches that are most likely to inhibit the cancer's growth or cause cell death.

Technologies Used:

•	Next-Generation Sequencing (NGS): NGS allows for comprehensive profiling of cancer genomes, identifying mutations in genes that drive cancer growth.

•	Liquid Biopsies: These tests analyse circulating tumour DNA (ctDNA) or other biomarkers in blood or other body fluids to detect genetic alterations and monitor treatment response.

•	Tissue Biopsies: Biopsy samples of tumour tissue are analysed to identify specific mutations or biomarkers.

Precision medicine enables the use of targeted therapies that block specific molecular pathways or cellular processes critical to cancer cell survival. Examples include:

•	EGFR Inhibitors: Used in non-small cell lung cancer (NSCLC) with EGFR mutations.

•	BRAF Inhibitors: Effective in melanoma with BRAF V600 mutations.

Immunotherapy: Biomarkers such as PD-L1 expression can guide the use of immune checkpoint inhibitors, which enhance the immune system's ability to recognise and attack cancer cells.

- PD-1/PD-L1 Inhibitors: Used across various cancers to unleash the immune response against tumours.

PARP Inhibitors: These drugs target cancers with deficiencies in DNA repair mechanisms, such as those with BRCA mutations in breast and ovarian cancers.

Combinatorial Approaches: Precision medicine allows for the combination of therapies based on genetic profiles to enhance treatment efficacy and overcome resistance mechanisms.

Genetic profiling facilitates participation in clinical trials testing new targeted therapies or combinations, expediting the advancement of innovative treatment options. Patients undergo genetic testing, which may involve procedures like tissue biopsies or liquid biopsies, to analyse the genetic characteristics of their cancer cells. Oncologists and molecular pathologists interpret this genetic data to identify actionable mutations or biomarkers that inform treatment decisions. Using the tumour's genetic profile, oncologists create a personalised treatment strategy that may incorporate targeted therapies, immunotherapies, or other precision medicine approaches. Throughout treatment, patients receive close monitoring to evaluate response and manage potential side effects. The treatment plan can be adjusted based on ongoing genetic testing and clinical assessments.

Precision medicine enhances treatment response rates and survival outcomes by focusing therapies on the specific genetic mutations that drive cancer growth. Unlike traditional chemotherapy, targeted therapies and other precision approaches typically result in fewer side effects because they pinpoint cancer cells more selectively. Each patient benefits from treatment customised to their individual genetic makeup, maximising effectiveness while minimising unnecessary treatments. Monitoring genetic changes during treatment enables early detection of resistance mechanisms, facilitating timely adjustments to preserve treatment efficacy.

Genetic testing and targeted therapies can incur high costs, with access often restricted by healthcare infrastructure and insurance coverage limitations. Cancers can mutate and evolve, necessitating continuous monitoring and adjustment of treatment approaches over time. It's essential to address concerns regarding data privacy, consent for genetic testing, and ensuring fair access to precision medicine.

Advancements in Precision Medicine

The field of precision medicine is rapidly evolving with ongoing advancements in genomic technologies, computational biology, and bioinformatics:

•	Liquid Biopsies: Advancements in detecting ctDNA and other biomarkers in blood samples are improving early cancer detection and monitoring treatment response.

•	Artificial Intelligence (AI): AI-driven algorithms are enhancing the analysis of complex genetic data, predicting treatment responses, and identifying new therapeutic targets.

•	Drug Development: Targeted therapies and immunotherapies continue to expand, with new drugs and combination therapies being developed based on genomic insights.

Precision medicine represents a paradigm shift in cancer treatment, offering personalised approaches based on the unique genetic profiles of individual patients. By targeting therapies to specific molecular alterations in cancer cells, precision medicine holds promise for improving treatment outcomes, reducing side effects, and advancing the field of oncology.

9. Clinical Trials: Participating in Experimental Treatments

Clinical trials are research studies conducted with human volunteers to evaluate new medical treatments, interventions, or devices. In oncology, clinical trials play a crucial role in advancing cancer care by testing the safety and efficacy of novel therapies, exploring new combinations of treatments, and improving understanding of cancer biology.

Clinical trials are essential for developing new treatments and improving existing therapies for cancer patients. They help translate scientific discoveries into practical applications that benefit patients. Experimental treatments tested in clinical trials include new drugs, targeted therapies, immunotherapies, and combination treatments aimed at improving outcomes and quality of life. Findings from clinical trials contribute to establishing new standards of care and treatment guidelines based on evidence-based medicine.

Types of Clinical Trials

Treatment Trials: Evaluate new drugs, therapies, or combinations of therapies aimed at treating cancer. These trials may compare new treatments with standard treatments or placebo.

Prevention Trials: Investigate ways to prevent cancer or reduce the risk of cancer recurrence, often involving lifestyle changes, medications, or vaccines.

Screening Trials: Focus on improving methods for detecting cancer early, when treatment is most effective.

Diagnostic Trials: Develop or improve tests and procedures for diagnosing cancer, such as imaging techniques or biomarker tests.

Phases of Clinical Trials

Phase I: Evaluate the safety, dosage, and potential side effects of a new treatment in a small group of patients. The primary goal is to determine the maximum tolerated dose (MTD) and identify side effects.

Phase II: Assess the effectiveness and further evaluate the safety of the treatment in a larger group of patients with specific types of cancer. These trials provide preliminary evidence of treatment efficacy.

Phase III: Compare the new treatment with the current standard treatment in a larger group of patients to determine superiority, non-inferiority, or equivalence in terms of efficacy and safety. Phase III trials are pivotal for gaining regulatory approval.

Phase IV: Conducted after a treatment has been approved and is on the market to further evaluate long-term safety, efficacy, and optimal use in broader patient populations.

Process of Participating in Clinical Trials

Patients must meet specific eligibility criteria based on factors such as cancer type, stage, prior treatments, and overall health to qualify for participation in a clinical trial. Before enrolment, they receive comprehensive information detailing the study's objectives, procedures, potential risks and benefits, and their rights as participants. Informed consent ensures that patients fully comprehend and willingly agree to participate. In randomised trials, patients may be randomly assigned to different treatment groups, whereas non-randomised trials assign treatments based on specific criteria. Throughout the trial, participants undergo regular monitoring, including medical exams, laboratory tests, imaging studies, and assessments of treatment response. Follow-up visits continue post-treatment to assess long-term outcomes.

Participants in clinical trials may access innovative treatments that are not yet widely accessible, potentially providing therapeutic advantages. They receive extensive medical attention, including ongoing monitoring and access to diverse teams of healthcare specialists. Engaging in trials allows patients to contribute to the progression of scientific understanding and the enhancement of future cancer therapies for broader benefits. Some trials also cover the expenses associated with investigational treatments, medical tests, and procedures, alleviating financial concerns for participants.

Experimental treatments may present unpredictable side effects or prove less efficacious compared to standard therapies. Participating involves a significant time commitment, requiring frequent visits to the study site and adherence to specific protocols, which may necessitate travel and time away from home. Safeguarding participant rights, privacy, and ensuring fully informed consent are paramount ethical considerations in clinical research.

Advancements and Future Directions

•	Precision Medicine Integration: Incorporating genetic profiling and biomarker testing into clinical trial design to personalise treatment strategies.

•	Immunotherapy Innovations: Developing novel immune-based therapies and combination approaches to enhance immune response against cancer.

•	Patient-Centered Research: Emphasising patient-reported outcomes and quality of life measures in clinical trial endpoints.

Clinical trials are essential for advancing cancer treatment, offering patients access to innovative therapies, contributing to scientific knowledge, and improving standards of care. By participating in clinical trials, patients play a pivotal role in shaping the future of cancer treatment and may benefit from promising new therapies not yet available outside of research settings. Through rigorous study protocols, ethical standards, and multidisciplinary collaboration, clinical trials continue to drive progress in oncology, providing hope and new possibilities for cancer patients worldwide.

10. Palliative Care: Managing Symptoms and Improving Quality of Life

Palliative care is a specialised medical approach focused on providing relief from the symptoms, pain, and stress of a serious illness, such as cancer. It aims to improve the quality of life for patients and their families through comprehensive care that addresses physical, emotional, social, and spiritual needs.

Palliative care considers the complete individual beyond their illness, concentrating on improving comfort and quality of life. It involves skilled management of symptoms like pain, nausea, fatigue, and shortness of breath to alleviate suffering. Palliative care also promotes transparent communication among patients, families, and healthcare providers regarding treatment goals, preferences, and end-of-life care decisions. Emotional, social, and spiritual needs are addressed through counselling, support groups, and spiritual guidance. Collaboration with the oncology team and other healthcare providers ensures coordinated and uninterrupted care.

Palliative care experts are skilled in employing advanced pain management techniques to ease troubling symptoms, enhancing comfort and well-being. By addressing the patient's physical, emotional, and social needs, palliative care improves quality of life throughout the cancer experience, regardless of the illness stage. It also provides crucial support to families and caregivers, offering guidance, education, and emotional assistance during difficult periods. Palliative care facilitates open and honest discussions about treatment options, prognosis, and care goals, empowering patients and families to make informed decisions.

It employs a blend of medications, interventions like nerve blocks, and integrative therapies such as acupuncture to effectively manage pain. Tailored treatment plans are utilised to address symptoms like nausea, vomiting, fatigue, shortness of breath, and loss of appetite. The program includes counselling, psychotherapy, and support groups to manage anxiety, depression, grief, and existential concerns. Spiritual guidance, rituals, and support are provided to patients and families, respecting their individual beliefs and values. Caregivers receive education and support to manage responsibilities, stress, and burnout. Additionally, the service assists with advance care planning, facilitating discussions about preferences for end-of-life care, hospice care, and comfort-focused interventions.

Early integration of palliative care alongside curative treatments, starting at the time of diagnosis, aims to manage symptoms and enhance quality of life. Palliative care specialists collaborate closely with oncologists and other healthcare providers to ensure seamless care and alignment of treatment goals. As the disease progresses or when aggressive treatments are no longer beneficial, palliative care may transition to hospice care, focusing on comfort and quality of life at the end of life. This approach prioritises patient and family preferences, values, and goals in decision-making, promoting dignity and autonomy throughout the care journey. Ongoing advancements in palliative care research and education contribute to improving practices and outcomes for cancer patients.

Palliative care is a critical component of comprehensive cancer care, focusing on symptom management, quality of life enhancement, and holistic support for patients and families facing serious illness. By integrating palliative care early in the cancer journey and aligning treatment with patient preferences, oncologists and palliative care specialists can optimise outcomes and provide compassionate, patient-centered care. As a fundamental aspect of modern oncology, palliative

Lifestyle and Holistic Approaches

11. Healthy Diet: Eating a Balanced Diet Rich in Fruits, Vegetables, and Whole Grains

A healthy diet plays a crucial role in cancer prevention, treatment, and overall well-being. It involves consuming a variety of nutrient-dense foods that support the body's immune system, promote healing, and reduce the risk of cancer recurrence.

Including a diverse array of fruits, vegetables, whole grains, lean proteins, and healthy fats in your diet ensures a rich supply of vital vitamins, minerals, antioxidants, and phytochemicals essential for overall health and immune function. Managing weight effectively through diet helps mitigate the risk of cancers linked to obesity and enhances treatment outcomes by fostering optimal bodily function. A well-balanced diet also fosters a healthy gut microbiome, crucial for regulating inflammation, supporting immune response, and facilitating nutrient absorption. Adequate nutrition boosts energy levels, bolsters resilience during cancer treatment, and enhances overall quality of life.

Specific Dietary Recommendations

Fruits and Vegetables: Rich in vitamins, minerals, and antioxidants (e.g., vitamin C, beta-carotene, lycopene), fruits and vegetables help protect cells from damage and support immune function. Aim for a variety of colours and types daily.

Whole Grains: Provide fibre, vitamins, and minerals essential for digestive health and overall well-being. Choose whole grains such as brown rice, quinoa, oats, and whole wheat bread over refined grains.

Lean Proteins: Include sources such as poultry, fish, beans, lentils, and tofu to support muscle strength, immune function, and tissue repair during cancer treatment.

Healthy Fats: Opt for unsaturated fats found in olive oil, avocados, nuts, and seeds, which promote heart health and provide essential fatty acids.

Hydration: Drink plenty of water throughout the day to maintain hydration and support cellular function. Limit sugary drinks and alcohol.

Evidence Supporting Diet in Cancer Care

Eating a diet abundant in fruits, vegetables, and whole grains has been linked to a lower risk of various cancers, such as colorectal, breast, and prostate cancers. Throughout cancer treatment, maintaining a balanced diet can aid in mitigating side effects like nausea, fatigue, and fluctuations in appetite. Essential nutrients such as vitamin D, vitamin C, zinc, and omega-3 fatty acids are critical for supporting immune function and may also lower the risk of infections during treatment. Antioxidants present in plant-based foods play a role in neutralising free radicals, which could potentially diminish cell damage associated with cancer initiation and progression.

Healthy Eating Strategies During Cancer Treatment

Individualised Approach: Consult with a registered dietitian or nutritionist to develop a personalised nutrition plan that meets your unique needs, preferences, and treatment goals.

Small, Frequent Meals: Eating smaller meals throughout the day may help manage nausea, improve digestion, and maintain energy levels.

Texture Modifications: Adjust food textures (e.g., pureed, soft, crunchy) based on swallowing difficulties or mouth sores caused by treatment.

Hydration: Stay hydrated with water, herbal teas, or broths to support kidney function and overall well-being.

Incorporating Holistic Approaches

Mindful Eating: Practice mindfulness during meals to savour flavours, textures, and nourishment, promoting relaxation and digestion.

Herbal Supplements: Discuss with your healthcare team before using herbal supplements, as they may interact with cancer treatments or medications.

Physical Activity: Combine a healthy diet with regular physical activity, as tolerated, to support overall health, reduce stress, and improve treatment outcomes.

A healthy diet rich in fruits, vegetables, and whole grains plays a vital role in cancer prevention, treatment support, and overall well-being. By nourishing the body with nutrient-dense foods and adopting healthy eating habits, individuals can optimise their nutritional status, enhance immune function, and improve quality of life during and after cancer treatment. Integrating dietary recommendations with holistic approaches and personalised care strategies empowers patients to actively participate in their health and well-being journey, fostering resilience and promoting long-term health outcomes.

12. Exercise: Regular Physical Activity to Improve Overall Health

Exercise is a fundamental component of a healthy lifestyle and plays a crucial role in cancer prevention, treatment support, and overall well-being. Incorporating regular physical activity into daily routines can positively impact physical function, mental health, treatment outcomes, and quality of life for cancer patients and survivors.

Regular physical activity contributes to maintaining and enhancing cardiovascular health, muscle strength, flexibility, and overall physical functioning. It also plays a crucial role in lowering the likelihood of chronic conditions such as diabetes and cardiovascular disease, which are particularly significant for individuals undergoing cancer treatment. Exercise supports mental clarity, reduces levels of stress, anxiety, and depression, and enhances mood and overall quality of life. Moreover, physical activity boosts immune function, potentially decreasing the susceptibility to infections during cancer treatment and aiding in recovery. Consistent exercise can combat the fatigue commonly associated with cancer treatment and improve overall energy levels. It also helps in managing weight, reducing body fat, and preserving muscle mass, all of which are essential for overall health and resilience during treatment. Activities like walking, jogging, and resistance training that involve bearing weight contribute to maintaining bone density and reducing the risk of osteoporosis.

Types of Exercise

Aerobic Exercise: Activities that increase heart rate and breathing, such as walking, jogging, swimming, cycling, dancing, and aerobic classes.

Strength Training: Exercises using resistance bands, free weights, or machines to build muscle strength and endurance.

Flexibility and Balance Exercises: Stretching, yoga, and tai chi improve flexibility, balance, and coordination, reducing the risk of falls and injuries.

Before initiating an exercise regimen, particularly during active treatment or recovery, it's crucial to consult healthcare professionals to ensure safety and suitability. Collaborate with oncologists, physical therapists, or exercise physiologists to create a tailored exercise program tailored to your specific cancer type, treatment plan, side effects, and overall fitness level. Begin with gentle activities and incrementally raise intensity and duration based on your tolerance and health condition. Modify exercise routines as needed to address treatment-related issues like fatigue, neuropathy, or joint discomfort.

Exercise Guidelines During Cancer Treatment

Frequency: Aim for at least 150 minutes of moderate-intensity aerobic exercise (e.g., brisk walking) or 75 minutes of vigorous-intensity exercise per week, spread across several days.

Intensity: Exercise at a level that raises heart rate and breathing rate but allows for conversation without difficulty.

Safety Precautions: Stay hydrated, wear appropriate clothing and footwear, and avoid exercising in extreme weather conditions or environments that may compromise health.

Benefits Across the Cancer Continuum

Prevention: Regular exercise may reduce the risk of developing certain types of cancer and other chronic diseases.

Treatment Support: Exercise can improve treatment tolerance, reduce side effects, and enhance recovery rates.

Survivorship: Maintaining regular physical activity after treatment can improve long-term health outcomes, reduce the risk of cancer recurrence, and enhance quality of life.

Combine exercise with other holistic approaches such as nutrition, stress management techniques (e.g., mindfulness, meditation), and supportive care services. Join exercise classes or support groups tailored for cancer survivors to enhance motivation, social support, and camaraderie.

Exercise is a powerful tool in cancer care, offering numerous physical, mental, and emotional benefits throughout the cancer journey. By incorporating regular physical activity into daily routines, cancer patients and survivors can optimise their health, improve treatment outcomes, and enhance overall quality of life. Collaborating with healthcare providers to develop personalised exercise plans and integrating exercise with holistic approaches promotes holistic well-being and empowers individuals to actively participate in their health and recovery.

13. Stress Management: Techniques like Yoga, Meditation, and Mindfulness

Stress management techniques such as yoga, meditation, and mindfulness play a pivotal role in supporting the overall well-being of individuals affected by cancer. These practices are integral components of holistic care, addressing not only psychological and emotional distress but also enhancing physical health and quality of life.

Yoga, meditation, and mindfulness foster relaxation, easing anxiety, alleviating depression, and bolstering emotional resilience throughout the challenges of cancer diagnosis and treatment. These practices are known to decrease blood pressure, lower heart rate, enhance sleep quality, and strengthen immune function, thereby supporting overall health and well-being. Mind-body techniques can also reduce the perception of pain and improve coping strategies for discomfort associated with cancer. By cultivating feelings of tranquillity, acceptance, and inner peace, these stress management methods improve quality of life and nurture a positive outlook.

Principles of Yoga, Meditation, and Mindfulness

Yoga: Combines physical postures (asanas), breathing exercises (pranayama), and meditation to improve flexibility, strength, balance, and mental clarity. Yoga classes tailored for cancer patients often emphasise gentle movements and relaxation techniques.

Meditation: Involves focusing attention and awareness on the present moment, often guided by breath awareness, visualisation, or mantra repetition. Meditation cultivates inner stillness, reduces stress, and enhances emotional well-being.

Mindfulness: Cultivates non-judgmental awareness of thoughts, emotions, and bodily sensations in the present moment. Mindfulness practices, such as mindful breathing or body scans, promote resilience, self-compassion, and stress reduction.

Types of Stress Management Techniques

Guided Imagery: Uses visualisation techniques to promote relaxation, reduce stress, and enhance healing. Imagery may involve imagining a peaceful place or visualising healing energy flowing through the body.

Breathwork: Focuses on conscious breathing techniques to regulate emotions, reduce anxiety, and induce a state of relaxation.

Progressive Muscle Relaxation: Involves tensing and then relaxing different muscle groups systematically to release physical tension and promote relaxation.

Tai Chi: An ancient Chinese martial art that combines slow, deliberate movements with deep breathing and meditation. Tai Chi enhances balance, flexibility, and mental focus, while promoting relaxation and stress relief.

Research shows that using stress management techniques can improve psychological health, reduce symptoms of anxiety and depression, and enhance the overall quality of life for cancer patients and survivors. Mindfulness-based practices, in particular, have been found to lower inflammation markers, boost immune function, and improve treatment tolerance.

Mind-body approaches can also support pain management by reducing pain perception and promoting relaxation. Integrating stress management techniques into comprehensive cancer care fosters holistic well-being by addressing the physical, emotional, and spiritual aspects of health. Oncology teams may recommend stress management programs, support groups, or integrative medicine services to enhance patient-centered care and overall treatment effectiveness. Learning and practicing these techniques empowers patients to take an active role in their healing journey, fostering self-care and resilience.

Stress management techniques such as yoga, meditation, and mindfulness are valuable tools in cancer care, offering profound benefits for patients and survivors. By reducing stress, promoting relaxation, and enhancing emotional well-being, these practices support overall health, treatment outcomes, and quality of life. Integrating stress management into comprehensive care plans empowers individuals to cultivate resilience, cope with the challenges of cancer, and foster a sense of inner peace and well-being.

14. Adequate Sleep: Ensuring Sufficient Rest and Sleep

Adequate sleep is essential for overall health and well-being, particularly for individuals navigating the challenges of cancer diagnosis, treatment, and recovery. Quality sleep supports immune function, cognitive function, emotional resilience, and physical recovery, making it a critical component of holistic cancer care.

Sleep is crucial for cellular repair, immune function, hormone regulation, and overall physical recovery, making it essential during cancer treatment. Quality sleep improves concentration, memory consolidation, and cognitive performance, aiding in maintaining mental clarity and decision-making abilities. Adequate sleep also enhances emotional resilience, reduces stress, anxiety, and irritability, promoting overall mood and emotional stability. Throughout cancer treatment, sufficient sleep supports recovery from surgeries, chemotherapy, radiation therapy, and other medical interventions, thereby optimising treatment outcomes.

Common Sleep Disturbances in Cancer Patients

Insomnia: Difficulty falling asleep, staying asleep, or waking up too early, often exacerbated by anxiety, pain, or treatment side effects.

Pain and Discomfort: Physical discomfort, such as pain, neuropathy, or surgical wounds, can disrupt sleep patterns and reduce sleep quality.

Medication Side Effects: Some cancer treatments and medications may cause insomnia, daytime drowsiness, or changes in sleep-wake cycles.

Emotional Distress: Stress, anxiety, depression, and uncertainty related to cancer diagnosis and treatment can lead to sleep disturbances.

Establishing a consistent sleep schedule involves going to bed and waking up at the same times every day, including weekends, to regulate your body's internal clock. Create a sleep-friendly environment by choosing a comfortable, quiet, and dimly lit space that encourages relaxation and supports restful sleep. Avoid consuming caffeine, nicotine, or heavy meals close to bedtime, as these can disrupt sleep quality and delay falling asleep. Incorporate calming bedtime rituals such as reading, gentle stretching, listening to soothing music, or practicing relaxation techniques to unwind before sleep. Follow recommended pain management strategies provided by healthcare professionals to alleviate discomfort and improve sleep quality.

Cognitive Behavioural Therapy for Insomnia (CBT-I) offers a structured approach to address thoughts, behaviours, and habits contributing to sleep difficulties, making it beneficial for managing chronic insomnia.

Quality sleep is crucial for supporting the immune system, which plays a vital role in combating infections and maintaining overall health during cancer treatment. Research indicates that improving sleep quality not only enhances the overall quality of life but also reduces fatigue and improves mood among cancer patients and survivors. Furthermore, adequate sleep can contribute to better treatment adherence, minimise treatment-related side effects, and improve recovery rates.

Various relaxation techniques, such as guided imagery, progressive muscle relaxation, or meditation, have been shown to promote relaxation and enhance sleep quality. Additionally, certain foods and herbal supplements are believed to support relaxation and sleep, although it's essential to seek guidance from healthcare providers before incorporating them into your routine. Complementary therapies like acupuncture, massage therapy, and aromatherapy are also options that can aid in promoting relaxation and maintaining good sleep hygiene.

Adequate sleep is a cornerstone of holistic cancer care, supporting physical health, cognitive function, emotional well-being, and overall quality of life. By prioritising sleep hygiene, managing sleep disturbances, and integrating relaxation techniques, cancer patients and survivors can optimise their recovery, treatment outcomes, and long-term health. Healthcare providers play a crucial role in addressing sleep-related issues, providing personalised strategies, and fostering comprehensive support to enhance sleep quality and promote overall well-being throughout the cancer journey.

15. Quit Smoking: Avoiding Tobacco Products

Quitting smoking and avoiding tobacco products are crucial steps in cancer prevention, treatment support, and overall health promotion. Tobacco use is a significant risk factor for various cancers and other chronic diseases, and cessation can lead to immediate and long-term health benefits.

Tobacco smoke contains numerous chemicals, including carcinogens that can harm DNA and heighten the likelihood of cancer. Ceasing smoking diminishes the risk of lung cancer, along with cancers affecting the mouth, throat, oesophagus, bladder, kidney, and pancreas. Smoking can impede the effectiveness of cancer treatments and elevate the chances of complications during surgeries, chemotherapy, radiation therapy, and other medical procedures. Quitting smoking enhances treatment outcomes and bolsters the body's healing capacity. For cancer survivors, quitting smoking reduces the risk of cancer recurrence and enhances long-term survival rates. It also lowers the risk of heart disease, stroke, lung disease, and other ailments linked to tobacco use, thereby fostering improved overall health and extending longevity.

Strategies for Tobacco Cessation

Behavioural Support: Engage in counselling, support groups, or smoking cessation programs that provide education, encouragement, and strategies to quit smoking.

Nicotine Replacement Therapy (NRT): Use nicotine patches, gum, lozenges, inhalers, or nasal sprays to reduce withdrawal symptoms and cravings.

Prescription Medications: Talk to healthcare providers about prescription medications such as bupropion (Zyban) or varenicline (Chantix), which can help reduce cravings and withdrawal symptoms.

Combination Therapies: Combine behavioural support with NRT or prescription medications for increased success in quitting smoking.

Support System: Inform family members, friends, and healthcare providers about your decision to quit smoking and seek their support in maintaining motivation and accountability.

Benefits of Quitting Smoking

After quitting smoking, lung function typically improves, and symptoms like coughing and shortness of breath diminish within a matter of weeks to months. Quitting also reduces the long-term risk of developing tobacco-related cancers and other chronic diseases.

In terms of cardiovascular health, quitting smoking leads to improvements in blood pressure, heart rate, and circulation, thereby lowering the risk of heart disease and stroke. Quitting smoking also enhances the effectiveness of cancer treatments and decreases the likelihood of complications during surgical procedures and recovery.

Moreover, quitting smoking results in financial savings by eliminating expenses previously allocated to tobacco products and reducing healthcare costs associated with smoking-related illnesses.

Research indicates that stopping smoking following a cancer diagnosis enhances survival rates and lowers the likelihood of cancer recurrence compared to continuing smoking. Non-smokers or those who have quit smoking typically endure cancer treatments more effectively, experiencing fewer complications and achieving better overall health outcomes. Ceasing smoking leads to significant long-term health advantages, improving quality of life and lessening the impact of chronic diseases.

Quitting smoking and avoiding tobacco products are pivotal steps in cancer prevention, treatment support, and overall health promotion. By committing to tobacco cessation, individuals can reduce their risk of cancer, improve treatment outcomes, enhance overall health, and increase longevity. Healthcare providers play a crucial role in supporting tobacco cessation efforts, providing resources, counselling, and personalised strategies to help patients and survivors quit smoking successfully. As part of comprehensive cancer care, prioritising tobacco cessation contributes to a healthier community, reduces healthcare costs, and promotes resilience and well-being among individuals affected by cancer.

16. Limit Alcohol: Reducing Alcohol Intake

Limiting alcohol consumption is essential for cancer prevention, treatment support, and overall health. Excessive alcohol use is a known risk factor for several types of cancer, including cancers of the mouth, throat, oesophagus, liver, breast, and colon. By reducing alcohol intake, individuals can lower their cancer risk, support treatment effectiveness, and improve overall well-being.

Drinking alcohol significantly increases the risk of developing several types of cancer, particularly when consumed excessively over an extended period. To reduce this risk and promote overall well-being, it's crucial to moderate alcohol intake. Excessive alcohol consumption can not only hinder the effectiveness of cancer treatments but also exacerbate treatment side effects and impair recovery rates. Therefore, limiting alcohol intake is essential for improving treatment outcomes and supporting the body's healing process.

The liver metabolises alcohol, and excessive consumption can lead to liver damage, inflammation, and an elevated risk of liver cancer. Cutting back on alcohol also lowers the risk of heart disease, hypertension, and other cardiovascular conditions, thereby enhancing overall health. For those who choose to drink alcohol, moderation is key. Moderate drinking is generally defined as consuming up to one drink per day for women and up to two drinks per day for men.

Individuals with a history of alcohol use disorder, liver disease, or specific medical conditions may benefit from abstaining from alcohol entirely. It is especially important for pregnant women and those planning pregnancy to avoid alcohol completely to prevent foetal alcohol spectrum disorders and other complications associated with pregnancy. Making informed choices about alcohol consumption supports better health outcomes and reduces the risk of alcohol-related health problems.

Strategies for Reducing Alcohol Consumption

Set Limits: Establish personal limits for alcohol consumption and stick to them. Keep track of drinks consumed and consider alternative beverages when socialising.

Behavioural Changes: Identify triggers for drinking and develop strategies to manage stress, social situations, and emotions without alcohol.

Seek Support: Talk to healthcare providers, counsellors, or support groups for guidance and encouragement in reducing alcohol consumption.

Substitute with Healthier Alternatives: Choose non-alcoholic beverages such as water, herbal teas, or sparkling water flavoured with fruit to reduce overall alcohol intake.

Research has demonstrated that reducing alcohol consumption significantly lowers the risk of alcohol-related cancers, such as those affecting the mouth, throat, liver, breast, and colon. Moderate alcohol intake supports liver health by reducing inflammation and decreasing the likelihood of liver disease and associated complications. For cancer patients undergoing treatment, limiting alcohol consumption can potentially improve tolerance to therapies, alleviate treatment-related side effects, and facilitate a smoother recovery process.

In addition to supporting liver function, reducing alcohol intake is beneficial for cardiovascular health, strengthens immune function, and reduces the risk of chronic diseases. Numerous scientific studies consistently link excessive alcohol consumption with an increased risk of developing specific types of cancer. By moderating alcohol consumption, individuals not only decrease these risks but also enhance overall health outcomes.

Limiting alcohol intake plays a crucial role in optimising the effectiveness of cancer treatments, minimising potential complications associated with therapy, and ultimately improving the overall quality of life for both cancer patients undergoing treatment and survivors. Making informed choices about alcohol consumption can significantly contribute to better health outcomes and well-being throughout the cancer journey.

Individuals with a history of alcohol use disorder, liver disease, or specific medical conditions may benefit from abstaining from alcohol entirely. It is especially important for pregnant women and those planning pregnancy to avoid alcohol completely to prevent fetal alcohol spectrum disorders and other complications associated with pregnancy. Making informed choices about alcohol consumption supports better health outcomes and reduces the risk of alcohol-related health problems.

Limiting alcohol consumption is integral to cancer prevention, treatment support, and overall health promotion. By reducing alcohol intake, individuals can lower their risk of alcohol-related cancers, support treatment effectiveness, and improve overall well-being. Healthcare providers, community organisations, and individuals all play a role in

17. Hydration: Drinking Plenty of Water

Hydration, or drinking plenty of water, is essential for overall health, especially for individuals undergoing cancer treatment or in recovery. Proper hydration supports bodily functions, aids in the management of treatment side effects, and contributes to overall well-being.

Water is crucial for cellular processes, nutrient transportation, and waste elimination throughout the body. Proper hydration ensures optimal organ function and overall physiological balance. Staying well-hydrated can help alleviate treatment side effects like nausea, fatigue, constipation, and dry mouth, which are common during cancer therapy. Additionally, water assists in flushing out toxins, supporting liver and kidney function, and promoting overall detoxification. Hydration also regulates body temperature, preventing overheating and maintaining thermal balance.

Proper hydration improves physical performance, muscle function, and endurance, which are vital for daily activities and exercise tolerance. Dehydration can negatively affect cognitive function, mood, and concentration, so drinking enough water supports mental clarity and cognitive health. Maintaining adequate hydration also enhances skin elasticity, moisture balance, and complexion, contributing to overall skin health and appearance. Additionally, water aids digestion, prevents constipation, and supports gastrointestinal function, which is especially important during cancer treatment when digestive issues may occur.

Tips for Staying Hydrated

Drink Throughout the Day: Sip water consistently throughout the day rather than consuming large amounts at once to maintain hydration levels.

Monitor Urine Colour: Check urine colour; pale yellow or clear urine generally indicates adequate hydration.

Hydrating Foods: Consume water-rich foods such as fruits (e.g., watermelon, oranges), vegetables (e.g., cucumber, celery), and soups to supplement fluid intake.

Limit Caffeine and Alcohol: Both caffeine and alcohol can contribute to dehydration, so consume them in moderation and balance with water intake.

Carry a Water Bottle: Keep a reusable water bottle handy as a reminder to drink water regularly, whether at home, work, or during outings.

Evidence Supporting Adequate Hydration in Cancer Care

Staying properly hydrated helps improve treatment tolerance, reduce fatigue, and enhance recovery from cancer therapies like chemotherapy and radiation. Sufficient water intake can alleviate treatment-related side effects such as nausea, constipation, and dry mouth, thereby enhancing overall comfort and quality of life. Hydration also supports immune function by maintaining adequate blood volume and lymphatic circulation, which are crucial for an effective immune response and overall health.

Integrative Approaches

Herbal teas like chamomile, ginger, or peppermint not only provide hydration but also offer additional health benefits, such as soothing digestive discomfort and promoting relaxation. During intense physical activity or illness, electrolyte-rich drinks or oral rehydration solutions can help maintain proper hydration and electrolyte balance.

Hydration is a fundamental aspect of holistic cancer care, supporting physical function, treatment tolerance, and overall well-being. By prioritising adequate fluid intake through water and hydrating foods, individuals can optimise their health, enhance treatment outcomes, and improve quality of life during and after cancer treatment. Healthcare providers play a crucial role in educating patients about the importance of hydration, monitoring fluid status, and providing personalised recommendations to support optimal hydration throughout the cancer journey.

18. Sun Protection: Using Sunscreen to Protect Against Skin Cancer

Sun protection is crucial for preventing skin cancer and maintaining skin health, especially for individuals at risk or undergoing cancer treatment. Exposure to ultraviolet (UV) radiation from the sun is a primary risk factor for skin cancer, including basal cell carcinoma, squamous cell carcinoma, and melanoma.

UV radiation damages the DNA in skin cells, heightening the risk of skin cancer over time. Implementing sun protection measures can reduce this risk and promote healthier skin. Sun exposure also contributes to premature aging, wrinkles, sunspots, and other signs of skin damage. Sun protection helps preserve a youthful skin appearance and texture. Additionally, certain cancer treatments like chemotherapy and radiation therapy can increase the skin's sensitivity to UV radiation. Therefore, sun protection is crucial to prevent further skin damage during treatment.

Methods for UV Radiation Protection

Sunscreen: Use broad-spectrum sunscreen with SPF (sun protection factor) 30 or higher. Apply generously to all exposed skin and reapply every two hours or after swimming or sweating.

Protective Clothing: Wear tightly woven clothing that covers arms, legs, and torso. Choose hats with wide brims to shade the face, ears, and neck.

Sunglasses: Wear UV-blocking sunglasses to protect eyes and the delicate skin around them from UV damage.

Seek Shade: Limit direct sun exposure during peak UV hours (10 a.m. to 4 p.m.) by staying in shaded areas, especially in sunny or high-altitude environments.

Benefits of Sunscreen Use

Consistent use of sunscreen lowers the risk of skin cancers, including melanoma, by blocking harmful UV radiation that damages skin cells. Sunscreen also helps prevent sun-induced wrinkles, age spots, and loss of skin elasticity, maintaining a youthful appearance. Additionally, whether for work or recreation, sunscreen protects against sunburn and cumulative UV damage during prolonged outdoor activities.

Research indicates that consistent use of sunscreen significantly reduces the occurrence of skin cancers, particularly among individuals with fair skin, a history of sunburns, or a family history of skin cancer. Sun protection measures are also crucial for minimising skin reactions and photosensitivity related to cancer treatments like chemotherapy and targeted therapies. Healthcare professionals play a vital role in educating patients about the importance of sun protection, the risks associated with skin cancer, and the proper application of sunscreen. They provide personalised guidance based on individual risk factors, skin type, and specific cancer treatment plans to ensure effective sun protection strategies are implemented.

Sun protection through the regular use of sunscreen and other measures is essential for preventing skin cancer, preserving skin health, and supporting individuals during cancer treatment. By integrating sun protection practices into daily routines and outdoor activities, individuals can reduce their risk of skin cancer, maintain skin integrity, and support overall well-being.

19. Regular Checkups: Frequent Health Screenings and Doctor Visits

Regular checkups and health screenings are essential components of proactive healthcare management, particularly for individuals at risk of cancer or undergoing cancer treatment. These routine appointments help detect health issues early, monitor treatment outcomes, and promote overall well-being.

Regular checkups enable early detection of health issues, including cancer and other chronic conditions, making treatment more effective. Healthcare providers evaluate overall health, review treatment plans, monitor for side effects, and adjust interventions as necessary during cancer treatment and survivorship. Routine screenings, vaccinations, and lifestyle counselling provided during checkups help prevent diseases and promote healthy habits.

Recommended Screenings

Depending on age, sex, and risk factors, screenings may include mammograms for breast cancer, Pap smears for cervical cancer, colonoscopies for colorectal cancer, and PSA tests for prostate cancer. Additional screenings such as blood pressure checks, cholesterol tests, blood glucose monitoring, and BMI assessments help detect cardiovascular disease, diabetes, and obesity-related complications. Early detection often leads to more successful treatment outcomes, reduced treatment intensity, and improved quality of life. Detecting cancers at early stages, when they are more treatable, can significantly lower mortality rates and increase survival chances. Early-stage cancers may require less aggressive treatments, preserving organ function and minimising side effects.

Research consistently shows that individuals who engage in regular health screenings experience higher survival rates and better health outcomes than those who do not undergo routine checkups. The practice of regular monitoring allows for early detection and intervention, which in turn improves quality of life by promptly addressing health issues, effectively managing symptoms, and promoting overall well-being. These screenings are critical in identifying potential health concerns at early stages when treatment is often more successful, highlighting the importance of proactive healthcare and regular check-ins with healthcare providers.

Regular checkups and health screenings are fundamental components of comprehensive cancer care, supporting early detection, effective treatment, and overall well-being. By prioritising routine health monitoring, individuals can detect health issues early, optimise treatment outcomes, and promote long-term health and resilience.

20. Support Groups: Joining Cancer Support Groups for Emotional Support

Joining cancer support groups can provide valuable emotional, practical, and social support for individuals and families affected by cancer. These groups offer a safe space to share experiences, receive encouragement, and access resources that promote well-being during and after cancer treatment.

Coping with cancer triggers a spectrum of emotions like fear, anxiety, sadness, and anger. Support groups provide a nurturing space where individuals can openly share their feelings, receive empathy, and find comfort in others who relate to their journey. Members share practical guidance, healthcare tips, and strategies for coping with treatment side effects, navigating the healthcare system, and accessing community support. By joining these groups, individuals cultivate a sense of belonging and diminish the isolation often felt with a cancer diagnosis. Many participants forge lasting friendships and supportive connections that endure well beyond the group sessions.

Group members in cancer support groups provide each other with mutual encouragement, empathy, and validation, which effectively combat feelings of loneliness and bolster emotional resilience. Discussions within these groups often revolve around practical strategies for managing treatment schedules, coping with treatment side effects, and navigating the daily challenges of cancer treatment and recovery. Additionally, guest speakers such as healthcare providers and specialists contribute valuable insights on topics ranging from nutrition and physical activity to stress management and complementary therapies. Studies indicate that participation in support groups significantly enhances psychosocial well-being by reducing distress and improving coping mechanisms among cancer patients and survivors. Being actively involved in these groups correlates with a higher quality of life, increased emotional stability, and improved adjustment to life changes following a cancer diagnosis. Throughout survivorship, involvement in support groups continues to play a crucial role by fostering resilience, strengthening social support networks, and aiding in the transition to post-treatment life. Through shared experiences and peer support, group members acquire effective coping strategies, develop problem-solving skills, and learn techniques to enhance their resilience and overall well-being.

Facilitating Support Group Participation

Finding Local Groups: Contact hospitals, cancer centres, community organisations, or online platforms to locate cancer-specific support groups in your area.

Online Resources: Virtual support groups offer flexibility for individuals who prefer online interactions or live in remote areas, providing access to peer support and educational resources.

Family and Caregiver Support: Some groups include sessions or separate groups for family members and caregivers, addressing their unique challenges and providing mutual support.

Joining cancer support groups offers invaluable emotional, practical, and social support for individuals and families navigating the challenges of cancer diagnosis, treatment, and survivorship. By participating in these groups, individuals can find solace, gain knowledge, build resilience, and forge meaningful connections with others who share similar experiences.

Complementary and Alternative Therapies

21. Acupuncture: For Pain and Symptom Management

Acupuncture is a centuries-old practice rooted in traditional Chinese medicine, increasingly recognised for its role in enhancing the quality of life for cancer patients and survivors. This therapeutic approach involves the insertion of thin needles into specific points on the body, aiming to restore the flow of vital energy (qi) and promote healing. While primarily known for pain management, acupuncture offers a range of benefits in alleviating symptoms associated with cancer and its treatments.

Acupuncture is believed to work by stimulating nerves, muscles, and connective tissues, promoting the release of endorphins (natural painkillers) and activating the body's own healing response. This stimulation helps regulate the nervous system, improve blood circulation, and enhance immune function, which are crucial for supporting overall health during cancer treatment.

One of the most well-documented benefits of acupuncture is its effectiveness in reducing pain intensity and enhancing pain management strategies. Cancer patients frequently suffer pain from the disease, surgical procedures, chemotherapy-induced neuropathy, or radiation therapy. Acupuncture can alleviate both acute and chronic pain, providing a non-pharmacological option for pain relief. Beyond pain relief, acupuncture is effective in managing a variety of cancer-related symptoms:

•	Nausea and Vomiting: Acupuncture has been shown to reduce chemotherapy-induced nausea and vomiting, providing relief and improving treatment adherence.

•	Fatigue: Cancer-related fatigue is a common and debilitating symptom. Acupuncture sessions can help alleviate fatigue, improve energy levels, and enhance overall vitality.

•	Insomnia: Many cancer patients struggle with sleep disturbances. Acupuncture promotes relaxation, reduces insomnia, and supports better sleep quality.

•	Anxiety and Depression: Cancer diagnosis and treatment often lead to heightened emotional distress. Acupuncture sessions promote relaxation, reduce anxiety, and improve mood, offering psychological support during a challenging time.

Safety and Considerations

Acupuncture is generally safe when performed by a qualified practitioner using sterile needles and following proper hygiene practices. It is crucial for cancer patients to seek an acupuncturist who has experience in treating individuals with cancer, as they can tailor treatments to address specific symptoms and health concerns.

Acupuncture serves as a complementary therapy that complements conventional cancer treatments like surgery, chemotherapy, and radiation therapy, rather than replacing standard medical care. It enhances treatment outcomes by promoting overall well-being, alleviating treatment-related side effects, and enhancing quality of life. Each acupuncture session is tailored to address the specific needs of the patient, taking into account factors such as cancer type, treatment stage, symptoms, and overall health status. This personalised approach ensures that acupuncture integrates smoothly with other aspects of cancer care, offering supportive benefits throughout the patient's healing journey.

Numerous clinical studies and systematic reviews support the efficacy of acupuncture in managing cancer-related symptoms and improving quality of life for patients and survivors. Research indicates that acupuncture is well-tolerated, improves pain outcomes, reduces treatment side effects, and enhances emotional well-being.

Acupuncture offers a valuable therapeutic option for cancer patients seeking pain relief, symptom management, and enhanced quality of life throughout their treatment and recovery journey. By integrating acupuncture into comprehensive cancer care plans, healthcare providers can address the holistic needs of patients, promote healing, and support resilience. Emphasising the role of acupuncture in complementary and alternative therapies fosters a patient-centered approach to cancer care, enhancing well-being and optimising treatment outcomes for individuals affected by cancer.

22. Massage Therapy: To Relieve Stress and Pain

Massage therapy is a widely recognised complementary treatment that offers significant benefits for cancer patients, focusing on alleviating stress, reducing pain, and enhancing overall well-being. This therapeutic approach involves the manipulation of soft tissues through various techniques to promote relaxation, improve circulation, and relieve muscle tension.

Massage therapy is highly valued for its dual benefits in providing physical relief and emotional comfort to cancer patients throughout their treatment and recovery journeys. Through gentle touch and soothing techniques, massage promotes relaxation, reduces anxiety, and supports the body's natural healing processes. It proves effective in managing pain associated with cancer treatments like surgery, chemotherapy, and radiation therapy by alleviating muscle tension, easing joint stiffness, and improving flexibility, thereby enhancing overall comfort and pain relief. Beyond its physical benefits, massage therapy addresses the emotional toll of cancer diagnosis and treatment by reducing stress hormones such as cortisol, boosting mood through the release of endorphins, and fostering a general sense of well-being. Additionally, massage techniques stimulate blood circulation and lymphatic drainage, which can aid in reducing swelling (lymphedema) and enhancing the delivery of oxygen and nutrients to tissues, thereby supporting overall health and healing. Regular massage sessions contribute to improved sleep quality, increased energy levels, and heightened emotional resilience, ultimately enhancing the overall quality of life during and after cancer treatment.

Cancer patients should consult with their healthcare team before beginning massage therapy, particularly if they have had recent surgery or have medical conditions that could impact the safety of receiving a massage. It is important to seek out a licensed massage therapist experienced in working with cancer patients. These practitioners are trained to tailor massage techniques to the specific needs and health conditions of those undergoing cancer treatment.

Massage therapy is recognised as a complementary treatment that seamlessly integrates into conventional cancer care plans. It collaborates with standard medical treatments to improve pain management, alleviate side effects from therapies, and promote overall well-being. Each massage session is customised by therapists to meet the specific needs of the patient, taking into account factors like cancer type, treatment stage, symptoms, and overall health condition. This personalised approach ensures that massage therapy harmonises with other components of cancer treatment, supporting each patient's individual path to recovery.

Evidence Supporting Massage Therapy in Cancer Care

Numerous studies and clinical trials have demonstrated the efficacy of massage therapy in improving symptom management and quality of life for cancer patients and survivors:

•	Pain Relief: Research indicates that massage therapy reduces pain intensity, improves pain tolerance, and enhances overall comfort for individuals undergoing cancer treatments.

•	Stress Reduction: Studies show that regular massage sessions reduce anxiety, depression, and emotional distress, promoting relaxation and improving emotional well-being.

•	Quality of Life: Patients report improved sleep, increased energy levels, and enhanced physical functioning after receiving massage therapy, contributing to a better overall quality of life.

Massage therapy offers valuable therapeutic benefits for cancer patients seeking pain relief, stress reduction, and improved quality of life during their treatment and recovery journey. By incorporating massage into comprehensive cancer care plans, healthcare providers can address the holistic needs of patients, promote relaxation, and support emotional resilience. Emphasising the role of massage therapy in complementary and alternative therapies fosters a patient-centered approach to cancer care, enhancing well-being and optimising treatment outcomes for individuals affected by cancer.

23. Herbal Supplements: Consulting with a Healthcare Provider About Safe Options

Herbal supplements are natural products derived from plants or plant extracts that are used for medicinal purposes. In the context of cancer care, many patients explore herbal supplements as complementary therapies to support treatment outcomes and improve quality of life. However, it is essential to approach herbal supplements cautiously and under the guidance of a qualified healthcare provider.

Herbal supplements are frequently used to complement conventional cancer treatments, helping to alleviate symptoms such as fatigue, nausea, pain, and boosting the immune system. These supplements are valued for their potential antioxidant, anti-inflammatory, and immune-boosting properties, which may enhance overall health and well-being during cancer treatment and recovery. However, it's important to be aware of safety concerns. Herbal supplements can interact with medications, affect treatment efficacy, and pose risks for individuals with specific health conditions. Therefore, cancer patients should consult their healthcare team about the use of herbal supplements to ensure they are safe and compatible with ongoing treatments. Additionally, the quality and potency of herbal supplements can vary significantly, so it is advisable to choose supplements from reputable manufacturers that adhere to quality standards and undergo third-party testing for purity and potency. While some herbs have shown promise in preliminary studies for managing cancer symptoms, more research is needed to confirm their safety and efficacy as complementary therapies.

Commonly Used Herbal Supplements

Turmeric (Curcumin): Known for its anti-inflammatory properties, turmeric may help reduce inflammation and support immune function.

Ginger: Used to alleviate nausea and vomiting associated with chemotherapy and improve digestion.

Green Tea: Contains antioxidants that may support cellular health and provide mild stimulation.

Mushrooms (e.g., Reishi, Shiitake): Known for immune-modulating properties and potential anti-cancer effects in laboratory studies.

Consulting with a Healthcare Provider

Discuss the use of herbal supplements with a healthcare provider knowledgeable in integrative oncology. They can offer personalised recommendations based on your specific cancer type, treatment plan, and overall health. Healthcare providers can evaluate potential interactions between herbal supplements and prescribed medications, minimising risks and optimising treatment outcomes. Regular monitoring during cancer treatment ensures that any changes in health status or side effects related to herbal supplements are promptly addressed. Additionally, healthcare providers educate patients about the benefits, risks, and limitations of herbal supplements, empowering them to make informed decisions about their health.

Herbal supplements offer potential benefits as complementary therapies for cancer patients seeking symptom relief and support during treatment. By collaborating with healthcare providers and integrating herbal supplements into comprehensive cancer care plans, patients can optimise treatment outcomes, manage symptoms effectively, and enhance overall well-being. Emphasising informed decision-making and safety protocols ensures that herbal supplements are used responsibly and contribute positively to the holistic approach to cancer care.

24. Aromatherapy: Using Essential Oils to Improve Well-Being

Aromatherapy operates on the principle that aromatic compounds from essential oils can exert therapeutic effects when inhaled, absorbed through the skin, or diluted for topical application. These oils contain natural plant compounds that interact with the body's limbic system, influencing emotions, mood, and physiological responses. This complementary therapy has gained popularity in cancer care for its potential to alleviate symptoms, reduce stress, and enhance quality of life.

Benefits in Cancer Care

Symptom Management: Essential oils are used to manage symptoms commonly experienced during cancer treatment, such as pain, nausea, fatigue, anxiety, and depression.

Stress Reduction: Aromatherapy promotes relaxation, reduces stress hormones like cortisol, and induces a calming effect, supporting emotional resilience during the cancer journey.

Improved Sleep: Certain essential oils, such as lavender and chamomile, are known for their sedative properties, helping to improve sleep quality and alleviate insomnia.

Enhanced Quality of Life: Regular use of aromatherapy can contribute to improved overall well-being, increased comfort, and enhanced coping mechanisms during and after cancer treatment.

Safety Considerations

Essential oils are highly concentrated and should be diluted before applying them to the skin to prevent irritation or allergic reactions. Always follow recommended dilution ratios and guidelines from a qualified aromatherapist. Cancer patients should consult their healthcare team before starting aromatherapy, especially if they have underlying health conditions or are undergoing treatments that may interact with essential oils. Choose high-quality essential oils from reputable suppliers to ensure purity, potency, and safety. Look for organic oils that undergo third-party testing for quality assurance.

Popular Essential Oils Used in Aromatherapy

Lavender: Known for its calming and sedative effects, lavender oil promotes relaxation and helps alleviate anxiety and insomnia.

Peppermint: Offers pain relief, reduces nausea, and boosts energy levels, making it beneficial for managing treatment side effects like chemotherapy-induced nausea.

Frankincense: Supports immune function, reduces inflammation, and promotes relaxation and emotional balance.

Lemon: Provides a refreshing scent that uplifts mood, enhances mental clarity, and supports detoxification.

Practical Applications

Inhalation: Direct inhalation of essential oils through a diffuser or inhaler allows for easy absorption and immediate benefits for respiratory and emotional support.

Topical Application: Diluted essential oils can be applied to the skin through massage or added to bathwater to promote relaxation and alleviate muscle tension.

Room Diffusion: Using an essential oil diffuser disperses aromatic molecules into the air, creating a calming atmosphere and enhancing the therapeutic benefits of aromatherapy.

Aromatherapy offers cancer patients a gentle and effective complementary therapy to manage symptoms, reduce stress, and improve overall well-being. By incorporating aromatherapy into comprehensive cancer care plans under the guidance of healthcare providers and qualified aromatherapists, patients can enhance treatment outcomes, alleviate discomfort, and promote emotional resilience throughout their cancer journey. Emphasising safe practices, informed decision-making, and the therapeutic benefits of essential oils fosters a holistic approach to cancer care that supports the physical, emotional, and psychological needs of individuals affected by cancer.

25. Hypnotherapy: For Pain and Stress Relief

Hypnotherapy is a therapeutic technique that utilises guided relaxation, focused attention, and suggestive imagery to achieve a heightened state of awareness and focused concentration, commonly known as hypnosis. This complementary therapy has shown promise in cancer care for managing pain, reducing stress, alleviating treatment-related side effects, and promoting overall well-being.

Hypnotherapy techniques, such as guided imagery and suggestion, can help reduce the perception of pain, enhance pain tolerance, and relax tense muscles. This approach is particularly effective for managing chronic pain and discomfort associated with cancer treatments. By inducing deep relaxation, hypnotherapy lowers stress hormones like cortisol and promotes emotional balance. It empowers patients to develop coping strategies, manage anxiety, and improve overall mental well-being. Hypnotherapy can alleviate a range of cancer-related symptoms, including nausea, fatigue, insomnia, and hot flashes, by addressing the underlying psychological and physiological factors contributing to these issues. Patients who undergo hypnotherapy often report increased motivation, better treatment adherence, and an enhanced ability to cope with treatment-related challenges.

Considerations for Cancer Patients

Hypnotherapy should be conducted by a qualified hypnotherapist or healthcare professional trained in hypnosis techniques. They can tailor sessions to meet the specific needs, concerns, and treatment goals of cancer patients. As a complementary therapy, hypnotherapy works alongside standard cancer treatments such as surgery, chemotherapy, and radiation therapy, enhancing overall treatment outcomes and quality of life without replacing medical care. Each hypnotherapy session is personalised to address the patient's unique symptoms, concerns, and goals. Therapists collaborate with healthcare teams to ensure coordinated care and holistic support.

Research has substantiated the effectiveness of hypnotherapy in alleviating pain intensity, mitigating treatment side effects, and enhancing psychological well-being for cancer patients and survivors. Patients frequently attest to marked improvements in mood, quality of life, and emotional resilience after undergoing hypnotherapy sessions, underscoring its positive influence on overall psychosocial health. Hypnotherapy empowers patients by equipping them with self-management techniques, bolstering coping skills, and fostering sustained emotional and physical well-being throughout their cancer journey and beyond.

Hypnotherapy offers cancer patients a valuable therapeutic approach for pain management, stress reduction, and symptom control through guided relaxation and focused attention. By integrating hypnotherapy into comprehensive cancer care plans, healthcare providers can address the holistic needs of patients, enhance treatment outcomes, and promote resilience throughout the cancer journey.

26. Reiki: Energy Healing Practices

Reiki is a spiritual healing practice that originated in Japan in the early 20th century. It involves the channelling of universal life force energy through the practitioner's hands to promote physical, emotional, and spiritual healing. This gentle, non-invasive therapy has gained popularity in cancer care for its potential to reduce stress, alleviate pain, and enhance overall well-being.

Reiki is based on the belief that life force energy flows through all living beings and is essential for maintaining health and well-being. The practitioner acts as a conduit for this energy, placing their hands lightly on or near the patient's body to facilitate healing. Reiki sessions promote relaxation, balance energy centres (chakras), and support the body's natural ability to heal itself.

Reiki induces a deep state of relaxation, lowers stress hormones like cortisol, and fosters a sense of peace and well-being. It helps patients cope with the anxiety, fear, and emotional turmoil associated with a cancer diagnosis and treatment. Reiki promotes pain relief by relaxing tense muscles, enhancing blood circulation, and supporting the body's natural pain-relieving mechanisms. It complements conventional pain management strategies and may reduce the need for pain medications. Cancer patients often face significant emotional and spiritual challenges, and Reiki sessions offer emotional support, foster a sense of connection, and promote inner peace and acceptance throughout the cancer journey.

Reiki is a gentle and non-invasive therapy generally safe for cancer patients, including those receiving active treatment or in palliative care. It does not interfere with medical treatments but enhances overall well-being. Each Reiki session is personalised to meet the unique needs and preferences of the patient. Practitioners collaborate closely with healthcare teams to integrate Reiki into comprehensive cancer care plans. As a complementary therapy, Reiki works alongside standard cancer treatments like surgery, chemotherapy, and radiation therapy, supporting holistic healing by addressing physical, emotional, and spiritual aspects of wellness.

Evidence Supporting Reiki in Cancer Care

Numerous cancer patients describe experiencing subjective benefits from Reiki, such as decreased pain, better sleep quality, increased emotional strength, and an overall sense of well-being. Although empirical evidence backing Reiki's effectiveness in cancer care is still developing, initial studies indicate positive results in managing pain, reducing stress, and enhancing quality of life for cancer patients. Reiki encourages patient-centered care by encouraging individuals to take an active role in their healing journey, promoting empowerment, self-awareness, and relaxation techniques.

Reiki offers cancer patients a gentle and supportive healing practice that addresses physical discomfort, emotional distress, and spiritual well-being. By integrating Reiki into comprehensive cancer care plans under the guidance of healthcare providers, patients can experience enhanced symptom relief, reduced stress, and improved quality of life throughout their treatment and recovery journey.

27. Chiropractic Care: Adjustments to Improve Physical Function

Chiropractic care is a healthcare discipline that focuses on the diagnosis, treatment, and prevention of disorders related to the musculoskeletal system, particularly the spine. It involves manual adjustments and manipulations of the spine and other joints to improve alignment, mobility, and overall physical function. In cancer care, chiropractic care is utilised as a complementary therapy to alleviate pain, reduce discomfort, enhance mobility, and support overall well-being.

Chiropractic care is based on the principle that proper alignment of the musculoskeletal structure, particularly the spine, allows the body to heal itself without surgery or medication. Chiropractors use hands-on adjustments (manipulations) to restore joint mobility, alleviate pain, and improve overall function of the nervous system.

Cancer and its treatments often lead to musculoskeletal pain, stiffness, and discomfort. Chiropractic adjustments offer relief by easing nerve pressure, relaxing muscles, and triggering natural pain relief mechanisms. Patients undergoing cancer treatment may experience decreased mobility and stiffness from therapy or extended periods of rest. Chiropractic care aids in restoring joint function, enhancing flexibility, and improving mobility, which supports daily activities and overall quality of life. Consistent chiropractic sessions can enhance physical well-being, lessen fatigue, and boost energy levels, helping patients manage the challenges of cancer treatment and recovery more effectively.

Cancer patients should prioritise seeking chiropractic care from licensed and experienced practitioners who have specialised training in oncology chiropractic or treating cancer patients. These professionals can customise techniques and treatment plans to ensure safety and effectiveness. Chiropractors collaborate closely with oncologists and other healthcare providers to seamlessly integrate chiropractic care into comprehensive cancer treatment plans. This collaborative approach ensures coordinated care and addresses the holistic needs of patients. Each chiropractic session is personalised to address the individual needs and concerns of the patient. Chiropractors consider the patient's cancer diagnosis, treatment history, symptoms, and overall health status to deliver tailored care that supports their well-being.

Integration with Conventional Care

Chiropractic care is considered a complementary therapy that works alongside conventional cancer treatments, such as surgery, chemotherapy, and radiation therapy. It supports the body's natural healing process, enhances pain management strategies, and improves overall quality of life.

Evidence Supporting Chiropractic Care in Cancer Care

Pain Relief: Research suggests that chiropractic adjustments can effectively reduce musculoskeletal pain, improve spinal function, and enhance mobility in cancer patients undergoing treatment.

Quality of Life: Studies indicate that chiropractic care contributes to improved physical functioning, reduced pain severity, and enhanced well-being among cancer patients and survivors.

Patient Satisfaction: Many cancer patients report high satisfaction with chiropractic care, noting improvements in pain relief, mobility, and overall quality of life.

Chiropractic care offers cancer patients a non-invasive and holistic approach to managing pain, improving mobility, and enhancing overall well-being during treatment and recovery. By integrating chiropractic care into comprehensive cancer care plans under the guidance of healthcare providers, patients can experience reduced pain, improved physical function, and increased resilience throughout their cancer journey.

28. Homeopathy: Using Highly Diluted Substances for Treatment (Controversial and Not Scientifically Supported)

Homeopathy is a holistic system of medicine that originated in the late 18th century and is based on the principle of "like cures like" and the concept of ultra-diluted substances. It involves using highly diluted preparations derived from plants, minerals, or animals to stimulate the body's self-healing mechanisms. While some individuals advocate for its use in cancer care and other health conditions, homeopathy remains controversial and lacks scientific support for its efficacy.

Homeopathy is founded on two main principles:

1.   Like Cures Like: The principle that a substance that causes symptoms in a healthy person can cure similar

symptoms in a sick person when administered in highly diluted form.

2.   Law of Minimum Dose: The belief that the more a substance is diluted, the more potent its healing properties become. Homeopathic remedies are typically diluted to the point where no molecules of the original substance remain.

Application in Cancer Care

Some proponents of homeopathy suggest that it can support cancer treatment by stimulating the body's natural healing responses, reducing treatment side effects, and improving quality of life. Homeopathic remedies are sometimes used to address symptoms such as pain, nausea, fatigue, and emotional distress associated with cancer and its treatments.

Controversies Surrounding Homeopathy

Lack of Scientific Evidence: The fundamental principles of homeopathy contradict established scientific knowledge and principles of pharmacology. Most systematic reviews and meta-analyses of clinical trials have found insufficient evidence to support the efficacy of homeopathy beyond a placebo effect.

Safety Concerns: Due to the extreme dilution of homeopathic remedies, they are generally considered safe when used as directed. However, concerns arise when patients rely on homeopathy as a substitute for evidence-based cancer treatments, which can delay effective medical care and potentially worsen outcomes.

Regulatory Issues: The regulation of homeopathic products varies widely across countries, leading to inconsistencies in quality control, safety standards, and consumer protection.

Considerations for Cancer Patients

Cancer patients interested in homeopathy should consult their healthcare team to discuss potential benefits, risks, and interactions with conventional cancer treatments. Patients and caregivers should be aware of the limited scientific evidence supporting homeopathy for cancer treatment and make decisions based on reliable information and professional guidance. Homeopathy should not replace proven cancer therapies like surgery, chemotherapy, radiation therapy, or targeted therapies. Instead, it may be used as a complementary therapy to aid in symptom management and improve quality of life, when integrated into a treatment plan under the supervision of healthcare providers.

While homeopathy remains a controversial topic in cancer care and healthcare in general, its principles and use continue to be debated among practitioners, researchers, and patients. The lack of robust scientific evidence supporting its efficacy and safety in treating cancer underscores the importance of informed decision-making and collaboration with healthcare providers.

29. Naturopathy: Combining Natural Therapies with Conventional Medicine

Naturopathy is a holistic approach to healthcare that emphasises prevention, natural healing, and the use of traditional and complementary therapies to support the body's inherent ability to heal itself. In cancer care, naturopathic medicine is often integrated with conventional treatments to enhance overall well-being, manage treatment side effects, and support the immune system.

Naturopathic medicine is guided by the following principles:

1.   Healing Power of Nature: Naturopaths believe in the body's innate ability to heal itself when given the right conditions, such as proper nutrition, lifestyle changes, and natural therapies.

2.   Identify and Treat the Cause: Naturopaths aim to identify and address the underlying causes of illness rather than merely treating symptoms.

3.   First, Do No Harm: Naturopathic treatments are chosen to minimise the risk of harmful side effects and support the body's natural healing processes.

4.   Treat the Whole Person: Naturopaths consider the physical, mental, emotional, and spiritual aspects of a person when developing treatment plans.

5.   Doctor as Teacher: Naturopaths educate and empower patients to take an active role in their health and well-being.

Naturopathic approaches in cancer care emphasise the use of natural therapies to complement conventional treatments and promote overall well-being. This approach may involve nutritional counselling, herbal medicine, and lifestyle adjustments aimed at managing symptoms such as pain, nausea, fatigue, and insomnia. Additionally, naturopathic methods focus on enhancing the immune system to bolster the body's ability to manage cancer and its treatments effectively.

For cancer patients undergoing naturopathic care, it is essential to maintain close collaboration with their oncologists and healthcare providers. Naturopathic treatments should be viewed as complementary to conventional cancer therapies, not as replacements. While some naturopathic treatments have shown benefits in managing symptoms and providing supportive care, their effectiveness in treating cancer directly is not well-established by scientific evidence. Patients are encouraged to seek evidence-based information and engage in discussions with their healthcare team regarding potential benefits and risks. Naturopathic treatment plans are tailored to the patient's specific cancer diagnosis, treatment plan, overall health, and personal preferences.

Common Naturopathic Therapies

Encouraging a diet centered around whole foods, abundant in fruits, vegetables, and lean proteins, to bolster overall health and immunity. Utilising plant-based remedies like echinacea to strengthen the immune system or ginger to alleviate nausea. Introducing practices such as meditation, yoga, and mindfulness to diminish stress and foster emotional well-being. Incorporating hydrotherapy, therapeutic massage, and acupuncture to alleviate pain and encourage relaxation.

Naturopathy offers cancer patients a holistic approach to health and healing that integrates natural therapies with conventional cancer treatments. By addressing the physical, emotional, and spiritual aspects of well-being, naturopathic medicine supports overall quality of life, symptom management, and resilience during the cancer journey.

Collaboration between naturopathic practitioners and oncologists ensures coordinated care and enhances patient-centered treatment plans that prioritise safety, efficacy, and comprehensive support for individuals affected by cancer.

30. Traditional Chinese Medicine: Including Acupuncture and Herbal Remedies

Traditional Chinese Medicine (TCM) is a comprehensive system of healthcare that has been practiced for thousands of years in China and other parts of Asia. It encompasses various therapies, including acupuncture, herbal medicine, dietary therapy, massage (Tui Na), and mind-body practices (such as Tai Chi and Qi Gong). In cancer care, TCM is used to support conventional treatments, manage symptoms, promote overall well-being, and address the underlying imbalances that contribute to disease.

TCM is based on several fundamental principles:

1.   Qi (Energy) Flow: Qi flows through the body along pathways called meridians. Imbalances or blockages in Qi can lead to illness, and TCM aims to restore balance and promote the smooth flow of Qi.

2.   Yin and Yang: Yin and Yang represent opposite forces that are interconnected and interdependent. Health is achieved through the balance of Yin (cold, passive, feminine) and Yang (hot, active, masculine).

3.   Five Elements: TCM categorises the body and its functions into five elements (Wood, Fire, Earth, Metal,

Water), each associated with specific organs, emotions, and qualities. Imbalances among these elements can affect health.

4.   Holistic Approach: TCM views the body as a whole, interconnected system where physical, emotional, and spiritual aspects are integrated.

Traditional Chinese Medicine (TCM) is employed to alleviate cancer-related symptoms, including pain, nausea, fatigue, insomnia, and emotional distress. TCM therapies complement conventional cancer treatments by enhancing the immune system, reducing treatment side effects, and improving overall quality of life. Practitioners of TCM customise treatment plans to address each patient's unique symptom patterns, constitution, and underlying imbalances, ensuring a holistic and personalised approach to care.

Considerations for Cancer Patients

Cancer patients should communicate openly with their oncologists and healthcare providers about any Traditional Chinese Medicine (TCM) therapies they are undergoing. This collaboration ensures treatments are well-coordinated and do not conflict with conventional cancer therapies. It's crucial to seek TCM treatments from qualified practitioners who follow safety standards and have experience working with cancer patients. Herbal remedies should be obtained from reputable suppliers to guarantee quality and safety. While ongoing clinical research investigates TCM's role in cancer care, therapies such as acupuncture have demonstrated promising outcomes in symptom relief and supportive care. Patients are encouraged to discuss potential benefits and risks with their healthcare team to make informed decisions.

Common TCM Therapies

Acupuncture: Involves the insertion of thin needles at specific points on the body to stimulate Qi flow, relieve pain, reduce nausea, and improve overall well-being.

Herbal Medicine: Uses plant-based remedies, such as ginseng, astragalus, and turmeric, to support immune function, reduce inflammation, and manage symptoms.

Dietary Therapy: Emphasises a balanced diet tailored to individual constitution and specific health concerns to promote healing and support overall health.

Mind-Body Practices: Include Tai Chi, Qi Gong, and meditation to reduce stress, enhance relaxation, and improve energy flow.

Traditional Chinese Medicine offers cancer patients a holistic and personalised approach to health and healing that integrates ancient wisdom with modern healthcare practices. By addressing the root causes of illness, promoting balance, and supporting the body's natural healing processes, TCM enhances symptom management, quality of life, and resilience during the cancer journey. Collaboration between TCM practitioners and oncologists fosters comprehensive treatment plans that prioritise patient-centered care, safety, and the integration of evidence-based complementary therapies.

Psychological and Emotional Approaches

31. Counselling: Professional Mental Health Support

Counselling is a vital component of cancer care that provides professional mental health support to patients, caregivers, and families facing the challenges of a cancer diagnosis and treatment. It encompasses various therapeutic approaches aimed at addressing emotional distress, enhancing coping strategies, and improving overall well-being.

Cancer diagnosis and treatment can evoke a wide range of emotions, including fear, anxiety, sadness, anger, and uncertainty. Counselling offers a safe and supportive environment where individuals can express their feelings, gain insight into their emotions, and develop effective coping mechanisms. It provides an opportunity to address psychological distress, improve communication with healthcare providers, and navigate the complexities of cancer treatment and survivorship.

Benefits of Counselling

Counsellors offer empathetic listening and validate emotions, supporting patients and families in processing their feelings and reducing isolation. Counselling provides individuals with practical coping skills and strategies to effectively manage stress, anxiety, depression, and other emotional challenges related to cancer. By addressing emotional and psychological concerns, counselling can improve overall quality of life, foster resilience, and promote a sense of empowerment and control. Counsellors also assist family members and caregivers, helping them navigate their roles, cope with caregiver stress, and enhance family dynamics with valuable support.

Different Therapeutic Modalities

•	Cognitive-Behavioural Therapy (CBT): Focuses on identifying and changing negative thought patterns and behaviours that contribute to emotional distress.

•	Mindfulness-Based Approaches: Incorporates techniques such as mindfulness meditation to cultivate present-moment awareness, reduce stress, and promote emotional well-being.

•	Supportive Therapy: Provides emotional support, validation, and guidance in a non-directive manner, allowing patients to explore their emotions and experiences at their own pace.

•	Interpersonal Therapy (IPT): Focuses on improving communication and relationships, addressing role transitions, and managing grief and loss.

Counselling sessions are custom-tailored to meet the specific needs, concerns, and preferences of each patient, taking into account their cancer diagnosis, treatment plan, and personal circumstances. Integrated within comprehensive cancer care plans, counselling collaborates closely with oncologists, nurses, and other healthcare providers to address the holistic needs of patients. Patients can expect confidentiality and establish a trusting therapeutic relationship with their counsellor, ensuring a safe environment for open communication and emotional exploration. Counselling services should be easily accessible to patients at various stages of their cancer journey, whether within hospital settings, cancer centres, community mental health centres, or through telehealth platforms, ensuring widespread availability and support.

Counselling plays a pivotal role in promoting resilience, emotional health, and adaptive coping strategies in cancer patients and survivors. It empowers individuals to navigate challenges, foster a positive outlook, and maintain a sense of hope and well-being amidst the uncertainties of cancer diagnosis, treatment, and survivorship. By addressing psychological and emotional needs, counselling contributes to comprehensive cancer care that supports the whole person— body, mind, and spirit.

Counselling is a cornerstone of psychosocial care in cancer treatment, providing essential support, guidance, and resources to enhance emotional well-being, resilience, and quality of life. By integrating counselling into cancer care plans, healthcare providers promote holistic healing, empower patients and families, and foster a compassionate and supportive environment throughout the cancer journey.

32. Positive Thinking: Maintaining a Hopeful Outlook

Positive thinking, also known as optimism or positive psychology, is a mental attitude that emphasises maintaining a hopeful and constructive outlook on life, even in the face of challenges like a cancer diagnosis. It involves cultivating thoughts, beliefs, and attitudes that promote resilience, emotional well-being, and a proactive approach to managing difficulties. Maintaining an optimistic outlook can significantly impact how individuals cope with a cancer diagnosis and treatment, helping them approach their situation with resilience, adaptability, and empowerment. Positive thinking doesn't ignore the realities of cancer but rather enhances coping strategies and contributes to a more positive overall experience during the cancer journey.

This approach involves identifying and challenging negative thought patterns or cognitive distortions that lead to pessimism or hopelessness and replacing them with more realistic and positive thoughts. Cultivating a habit of acknowledging and appreciating the positive aspects of life, even in difficult times, can shift focus towards positivity. Keeping a gratitude journal or regularly reflecting on blessings can help achieve this mindset. Mindfulness meditation techniques promote present-moment awareness, reduce stress, and strengthen emotional resilience by emphasising acceptance and non-judgment of thoughts and emotions. Establishing reachable goals and milestones fosters a sense of purpose, accomplishment, and motivation, further contributing to a positive outlook.

Benefits for Patients

•   Enhanced Emotional Well-being: Positive thinking can reduce feelings of anxiety, fear, and depression commonly associated with a cancer diagnosis. It promotes emotional resilience and adaptive coping mechanisms.

- **Improved Quality of Life:** Maintaining a hopeful outlook can enhance overall quality of life by promoting a sense of control, empowerment, and well-being.

- **Better Treatment Adherence:** Patients who maintain a positive attitude may be more likely to adhere to their treatment plans, engage in self-care practices, and actively participate in their recovery.

Considerations

- **Balanced Perspective:** Positive thinking does not mean ignoring or denying negative emotions. It involves acknowledging and processing difficult feelings while actively cultivating a mindset that focuses on strengths, resilience, and opportunities for growth.

- **Individual Differences:** Coping styles vary among individuals, and what works for one person may not be effective for another. It's important for patients to explore different strategies and find approaches that resonate with their personal preferences and circumstances.

- **Support System:** Building a strong support network of family, friends, and healthcare providers who foster positivity and encouragement can reinforce the benefits of positive thinking.

Role in Promoting Overall Psychological Health

Positive thinking plays a crucial role in promoting psychological health and well-being throughout the cancer journey. It encourages patients to maintain a proactive and empowered approach to their health, fosters emotional resilience, and supports adaptive coping with challenges. By cultivating optimism and hope, individuals can navigate the uncertainties of cancer treatment with greater confidence, strength, and a sense of purpose.

Positive thinking is a powerful psychological approach that enhances emotional resilience, promotes adaptive coping strategies, and improves overall quality of life for cancer patients and survivors. By integrating strategies for fostering optimism into daily life and treatment plans, healthcare providers can support patients in cultivating a hopeful outlook that nurtures psychological well-being and facilitates a proactive approach to managing cancer and its impact.

33. Visualisation: Imagining the Body Healing

Visualisation, also known as guided imagery or mental imagery, is a powerful technique used in cancer care to promote relaxation, reduce stress, and enhance healing by harnessing the mind-body connection. It involves creating vivid mental images or scenarios that evoke positive sensations, emotions, and outcomes, such as the body's healing process.

Visualisation operates on the principle that the mind and body are interconnected, allowing mental imagery to influence physical and emotional states. By vividly imagining healing processes, individuals can stimulate physiological responses, promote relaxation, and support overall well-being. These techniques help alleviate stress, anxiety, and tension often associated with a cancer diagnosis, treatment, and uncertainty. By envisioning calming scenes or sensations, individuals can reduce their perception of pain and increase their overall comfort. Visualisation nurtures the body's innate healing mechanisms by cultivating a positive mental outlook and encouraging relaxation, offering a sense of control, empowerment, and hope during difficult times. This enhances emotional resilience and minimises feelings of helplessness. By redirecting focus and promoting relaxation, visualisation can complement pain management approaches and decrease dependence on pain medications. Patients often experience an improved quality of life, enhanced mood, and better management of treatment-related side effects through consistent practice of visualisation techniques.

Techniques for Practice

Listening to a recorded script or guidance that directs the visualisation process, often led by a healthcare professional or trained practitioner. Crafting personalised mental images or scenarios that evoke feelings of relaxation, healing, and overall well-being. Patients can practice visualisation independently or with the encouragement of loved ones. Involving multiple senses—sight, sound, touch, smell, and taste—in mental imagery to create a richer and more immersive experience. Consistent practice enhances the efficacy of visualisation techniques, strengthening positive mental states and fostering lasting benefits.

Visualisation techniques should be tailored to each patient's preferences, comfort level, and specific needs. These techniques complement conventional cancer treatments and other psychological and emotional support therapies, enhancing holistic patient care. Patients may benefit from guidance and support from healthcare providers or qualified practitioners experienced in using visualization techniques in cancer care. Visualisation empowers cancer patients to actively participate in their healing journey, promoting a sense of empowerment, hope, and control over their health. By cultivating positive mental imagery and emotional states, individuals can mitigate stress, enhance coping strategies, and support overall psychological well-being throughout treatment and recovery.

Visualisation is a valuable psychological approach in cancer care that harnesses the mind's power to promote relaxation, reduce stress, and enhance healing. Through vivid mental imagery and positive visualisation, patients can cultivate resilience, manage emotional challenges, and support their body's natural healing processes.

34. Creative Arts Therapy: Using Art, Music, or Dance for Expression and Healing

Creative arts therapy encompasses various modalities—including art therapy, music therapy, dance/movement therapy, and expressive writing—that utilise artistic expression to promote emotional healing, reduce stress, and enhance well-being in cancer patients and survivors. These therapies provide a creative outlet for self-expression, processing emotions, and fostering resilience amidst the challenges of cancer diagnosis and treatment.

Creative arts therapy is grounded in the belief that artistic expression can facilitate emotional healing and personal growth. It integrates creative processes with therapeutic principles to address psychological, emotional, and spiritual aspects of well-being. Creative arts therapy enables patients to explore and express complex emotions, fears, hopes, and challenges associated with their cancer journey. Participating in creative endeavours like artmaking, music listening, or dance/movement can reduce stress, foster relaxation, and enhance mood. In therapeutic environments, patients find a secure, non-judgmental space to pursue self-discovery, boost self-esteem, and connect with peers facing similar circumstances. Creative arts therapy provides a valuable outlet for navigating challenging emotions, alleviating anxiety, and facilitating emotional release. Engaging in creative expression allows patients to articulate thoughts and emotions that words alone may not fully convey. Involvement in creative arts activities can improve overall quality of life, instil a sense of purpose and achievement, and cultivate a positive perspective.

Techniques for Practice

•	Art Therapy: Using visual arts (painting, drawing, sculpture) to explore emotions, symbols, and narratives related to the cancer experience.

•	Music Therapy: Listening to music, creating music, or engaging in rhythmic activities to promote relaxation, emotional expression, and stress reduction.

•	Dance/Movement Therapy: Utilising movement, dance, and expressive gestures to embody emotions, release tension, and enhance body awareness.

•	Expressive Writing: Writing journals, poetry, or narratives to process thoughts and emotions, gain insights, and promote self-reflection.

Considerations

- Accessibility: Creative arts therapy should be accessible to patients of varying abilities and preferences, ensuring inclusivity and participation.

- Professional Guidance: Qualified therapists with training in creative arts modalities ensure safe, supportive, and effective therapeutic experiences.

- Integration with Care Plans: Creative arts therapies complement conventional cancer treatments and other psychosocial interventions, contributing to comprehensive patient-centered care.

Creative arts therapy empowers cancer patients to explore, express, and transform their cancer journey through creative expression. By engaging in artistic processes, individuals can foster resilience, cope with treatment-related challenges, and cultivate a deeper understanding of self and healing possibilities.

Creative arts therapy offers a transformative approach to emotional and psychological support in cancer care, utilising artistic expression to promote healing, reduce stress, and enhance well-being. Through art, music, dance, and writing, patients can access profound avenues for self-expression, emotional exploration, and personal growth amidst the complexities of cancer diagnosis and treatment.

35. Spiritual Practices: Engaging in Religious or Spiritual Activities

Spiritual practices encompass a wide range of religious and spiritual activities that provide comfort, solace, and a sense of connection to something greater than oneself. For cancer patients and survivors, these practices can offer profound support, inner strength, and a source of meaning and hope during challenging times.

Spiritual practices hold significant importance in cancer care, addressing the spiritual and existential dimensions of illness beyond physical health. They provide a framework for coping with uncertainty, finding meaning in suffering, and navigating existential questions related to life, death, and purpose.

Participating in spiritual practices can offer comfort, solace, and a profound sense of peace during challenging times throughout the cancer journey. These beliefs and practices provide patients with a framework for discovering meaning in their experiences, nurturing hope, and sustaining a positive perspective. Spiritual communities, rituals, and practices also offer emotional support, foster connections with others, and create opportunities for shared experiences and collective prayers.

Types of Spiritual Practices

Engaging in prayer for healing, guidance, strength, and peace, whether individually or as part of a community, offers comfort and a profound sense of connection. Practicing contemplative methods to still the mind, contemplate spiritual teachings, and foster inner peace and resilience. Participating in religious or spiritual rituals, such as ceremonies, sacraments, or rites, that commemorate significant milestones or offer spiritual guidance. Seeking solidarity and encouragement from religious or spiritual communities through attending services, group meetings, or spiritual retreats fosters fellowship and support.

Considerations

Spiritual practices should be tailored to reflect patients' personal beliefs, values, and cultural backgrounds, honouring their individual preferences and spiritual paths. Integration into Care: Healthcare providers should recognise and accommodate patients' spiritual needs as integral to comprehensive cancer care, collaborating with chaplains, counsellors, or spiritual advisors as necessary. Respect for Diversity: Embracing and honouring a variety of spiritual beliefs and practices, promoting inclusivity, and offering non-denominational support as required.

Spiritual practices play a crucial role in fostering resilience, promoting emotional well-being, and enhancing coping strategies in cancer patients. By nurturing spiritual connections, patients can draw strength from their beliefs, find peace amidst uncertainty, and cultivate a sense of hope and purpose in their journey towards healing and recovery.

Spiritual practices offer profound support and meaning in cancer care, addressing the spiritual and existential dimensions of illness. By engaging in prayer, meditation, rituals, and community support, patients can find comfort, solace, and a sense of connection to something greater than themselves. Integrating spiritual practices into comprehensive cancer care plans empowers patients to navigate challenges, find meaning in their experiences, and foster resilience, hope, and emotional well-being throughout their cancer journey.

Unconventional and Experimental Ideas

36. Cannabis Oil: Using CBD or THC for Symptom Management (Legal Status Varies)

Cannabis oil, derived from the cannabis plant, has gained attention for its potential therapeutic benefits in managing symptoms related to cancer and its treatment. It contains cannabinoids, including cannabidiol (CBD) and tetrahydrocannabinol (THC), which interact with the body's endocannabinoid system to potentially alleviate pain, nausea, and other side effects

Understanding Cannabis Oil

•	CBD vs. THC: Cannabis oil can be derived from marijuana plants containing varying levels of CBD and THC. CBD is non-psychoactive and is often used for pain relief, reducing inflammation, and managing anxiety without the "high" associated with THC. THC, on the other hand, is psychoactive and may help with pain, nausea, and appetite stimulation.

•	Endocannabinoid System: The body's endocannabinoid system plays a role in regulating various physiological processes, including pain sensation, mood, appetite, and immune function. Cannabinoids in cannabis oil interact with cannabinoid receptors in this system, potentially influencing these processes.

Legal Status

•	Varies by Region: The legal status of cannabis oil, CBD, and THC varies widely by country, state, and jurisdiction. Some regions have legalised medical cannabis, allowing patients to access cannabis products with a prescription or medical card. However, legal regulations often restrict cultivation, distribution, and possession of cannabis products.

•	Medical vs. Recreational Use: In places where medical cannabis is legal, patients may obtain cannabis oil through licensed dispensaries or healthcare providers. Recreational use of cannabis products, including cannabis oil, is subject to separate regulations and may not be legal in all areas.

Potential Benefits

Cannabis oil, especially formulations containing THC, has demonstrated potential in easing cancer-related pain by interacting with pain receptors in the nervous system. THC in cannabis oil shows promise in alleviating chemotherapy-induced nausea and vomiting, potentially enhancing appetite and overall quality of life. Additionally, CBD in cannabis oil may impart calming effects, helping to reduce anxiety and stress commonly faced by cancer patients. THC has also been linked to increased appetite, which can be advantageous for patients dealing with cancer-related appetite loss and weight reduction.

Considerations

Prior to exploring cannabis oil, patients should seek guidance from their healthcare provider, particularly oncologists or palliative care specialists knowledgeable about its potential advantages and risks in cancer treatment. Patients and caregivers should also be mindful of local laws and regulations governing the use of cannabis products, understanding legal implications and possible consequences. Obtaining cannabis oil from trustworthy sources ensures product integrity, purity, and precise cannabinoid composition. Quality assurance measures help minimise risks associated with contamination or inconsistencies in potency.

Cannabis oil represents an experimental approach to symptom management in cancer care, particularly for alleviating pain, nausea, and other treatment-related side effects. Research continues to explore its therapeutic potential, safety profile, and optimal use in complementary and integrative oncology.

Cannabis oil, containing CBD and THC, offers potential benefits for symptom management in cancer care, including pain relief, nausea reduction, and appetite stimulation. Its use as an experimental therapy requires careful consideration of legal, medical, and ethical factors. By consulting healthcare providers and adhering to legal regulations, patients can explore cannabis oil as part of a holistic approach to managing cancer symptoms and improving quality of life. Ongoing research and clinical trials contribute to understanding its role in cancer care, highlighting opportunities for further exploration and integration into comprehensive treatment plans.

37. Cryotherapy: Exposing the Body to Extremely Cold Temperatures

Cryotherapy involves exposing the body to extremely cold temperatures for therapeutic purposes. This approach has garnered interest in cancer treatment for its potential benefits in reducing side effects of chemotherapy, enhancing immune response, and targeting tumours.

Cryotherapy involves the application of cold temperatures to targeted areas of the body or the entire body, employing methods such as ice packs, cryochambers, or localised cryoprobes. Localised cryotherapy precisely targets specific areas like tumours or inflamed tissues with controlled cold application. Meanwhile, whole-body cryotherapy exposes the entire body to extreme cold in a controlled environment.

Cryotherapy has shown promise in alleviating chemotherapy side effects such as nausea, neuropathy, and inflammation by cooling the body before or after treatment. Additionally, cryotherapy can be used in cryoablation, where freezing temperatures delivered directly to tumours via probes induce cell death and shrink tumours. This technique has been effective in certain cases for destroying cancerous growths. Furthermore, exposure to cold has been demonstrated to boost the immune system, potentially enhancing the immune response against cancer cells and supporting overall immune function. Cryotherapy can effectively alleviate cancer-related pain by numbing nerve endings and reducing inflammation in affected areas, providing comfort to patients. Compared to traditional surgical methods, cryoablation is less invasive and may lead to shorter recovery times, reduced hospital stays, and fewer complications. Cryotherapy techniques focus on targeting cancerous tissues specifically while preserving nearby healthy tissues, thereby minimizing damage to adjacent organs or structures.

Not all patients are suitable candidates for cryotherapy, as factors like tumour size, location, and individual health conditions must be assessed by healthcare providers to determine suitability. Potential side effects may include skin irritation, numbness, and temporary discomfort during or after treatment, which typically resolve as the body readjusts to normal temperatures.

Integration with Treatment Plans: Cryotherapy is frequently used as a complementary therapy alongside conventional cancer treatments such as chemotherapy, radiation therapy, or surgery. Collaboration with oncologists and multidisciplinary teams ensures comprehensive patient care.

Role as an Experimental Approach

Cryotherapy represents an experimental approach in cancer care, particularly in managing treatment side effects, targeting tumours, and supporting immune function. Ongoing research and clinical trials continue to explore its efficacy, safety profile, and optimal integration into personalised treatment plans.

Cryotherapy offers potential benefits in cancer care through its ability to reduce chemotherapy side effects, target tumours, and stimulate immune response. As an experimental therapy, its application requires careful consideration of patient suitability, treatment goals, and integration with conventional treatments.

38. Hyperbaric Oxygen Therapy: Breathing Pure Oxygen in a Pressurised Room

Hyperbaric oxygen therapy (HBOT) involves breathing pure oxygen in a pressurised environment, typically in a hyperbaric chamber. This treatment has been explored in cancer care for its potential benefits in enhancing oxygen delivery to tissues, supporting wound healing, and possibly affecting tumour biology.

Hyperbaric oxygen therapy (HBOT) increases oxygen levels in the bloodstream and tissues by subjecting patients to elevated atmospheric pressure while they breathe pure oxygen. This process helps oxygen dissolve into body fluids and improves its distribution to cells. Hyperbaric chambers are designed to withstand these heightened pressure conditions, and patients typically undergo treatment sessions inside these chambers for 30 minutes to two hours, providing a comfortable environment for therapy. HBOT aims to boost oxygen levels in tissues, potentially aiding healing processes, enhancing immune function, and influencing the tumour microenvironment. It is used to alleviate radiation-induced tissue damage by promoting tissue repair, reducing inflammation, and aiding in the recovery of irradiated tissues. HBOT is often integrated as a complementary therapy with conventional cancer treatments like radiation therapy and surgery, aiming to maximize treatment effectiveness and improve overall quality of life.

Potential Benefits

•	Wound Healing: HBOT accelerates wound healing in patients with radiation-induced skin ulcers, surgical wounds, or tissue damage resulting from cancer treatments.

•	Radiation Therapy Side Effects: By reducing tissue hypoxia (oxygen deficiency), HBOT may minimise radiation therapy side effects, such as delayed wound healing and tissue necrosis.

•	Antitumor Effects: Research is ongoing to explore HBOT's potential direct effects on tumour biology, including oxygen sensitivity and tumour growth inhibition in certain cancers.

Healthcare providers assess the suitability of HBOT for patients by evaluating their medical history, current health status, and treatment goals. Considerations include lung function, ear health, and cardiovascular condition. Potential side effects of HBOT may include ear barotrauma, sinus discomfort, temporary vision changes, and, in rare cases, oxygen toxicity, though these effects are generally mild and short-lived. Collaboration with oncologists, radiation oncologists, and wound care specialists ensures comprehensive care and the integration of HBOT into personalised treatment strategies.

Role as an Experimental Approach

HBOT represents an experimental approach in cancer care, particularly in managing treatment side effects, supporting tissue recovery, and potentially influencing tumour biology. Ongoing research continues to investigate its efficacy, safety profile, and optimal integration into comprehensive cancer treatment strategies.

Hyperbaric oxygen therapy offers potential benefits in cancer care by enhancing tissue oxygenation, supporting wound healing, and potentially affecting tumour biology. As an experimental therapy, its application requires careful consideration of patient suitability, treatment objectives, and collaboration with healthcare providers.

39. Fasting: Periodic Fasting Under Medical Supervision

Fasting, the practice of abstaining from food for defined periods, has garnered attention in cancer research for its potential effects on metabolism, cellular repair mechanisms, and possibly enhancing the body's response to cancer treatment.

Fasting can be practiced in various ways, such as intermittent fasting (IF), where eating and fasting cycles alternate, or prolonged fasting lasting 24 hours or more. Mechanistically, fasting induces metabolic shifts like lowered blood sugar and insulin levels, heightened ketone body production, and activation of cellular repair mechanisms such as autophagy (cellular cleansing) and apoptosis (programmed cell death). Fasting has been explored for its potential to mitigate chemotherapy and radiation therapy side effects by safeguarding healthy cells and tissues while possibly sensitising cancer cells to treatment. It triggers metabolic changes that could impede cancer cell growth and proliferation, as cancer cells typically rely heavily on glucose for energy. Additionally, fasting might influence immune responses, potentially bolstering immune surveillance and the body's ability to combat cancer cells. Research in animal models indicates that fasting could heighten the sensitivity of cancer cells to chemotherapy and radiation therapy, potentially amplifying their therapeutic impact. Fasting has also shown promise in lowering inflammation markers, which could be advantageous for cancer patients dealing with persistent inflammation. Certain individuals have reported enhanced well-being, mental clarity, and increased energy levels while fasting, which may positively impact their overall quality of life.

Considerations

•	Medical Supervision: Fasting should be conducted under medical supervision, especially for cancer patients undergoing active treatment or with specific medical conditions that may affect fasting tolerance.

•	Individualised Approach: The duration and type of fasting should be tailored to individual patient needs, considering factors such as cancer type, treatment stage, nutritional status, and overall health.

•	Nutritional Support: Adequate hydration and nutritional support before and after fasting periods are essential to maintain hydration, electrolyte balance, and prevent nutritional deficiencies.

Fasting represents an experimental approach in cancer care, exploring its potential effects on treatment outcomes, metabolic health, and overall well-being. Ongoing research aims to elucidate its mechanisms of action, optimise fasting protocols, and evaluate its safety and efficacy in different cancer types and patient populations.

Fasting holds promise as an experimental strategy in cancer care, leveraging metabolic changes and potential synergies with conventional treatments to enhance therapeutic outcomes. As research progresses, understanding the impact of fasting on cancer metabolism, treatment tolerance, and patient well-being continues to evolve.

40. Keto Diet: High-Fat, Low-Carb Diet to Starve Cancer Cells

The ketogenic diet, or keto diet, is a high-fat, low-carbohydrate dietary approach that has gained attention in cancer research for its potential to starve cancer cells by altering metabolism and reducing glucose availability.

Understanding the Keto Diet

•	Macronutrient Composition: The keto diet emphasises high fat (typically 70-80% of total calories), moderate protein (20-25%), and very low carbohydrate intake (usually less than 50 grams per day). This dietary composition induces a metabolic state known as ketosis, where the body produces ketone bodies from fats for energy instead of glucose.

•	Metabolic Changes: Ketosis shifts the body's primary fuel source from glucose to fats and ketones. This metabolic switch may inhibit cancer cell growth, as many cancer cells rely heavily on glucose (sugar) for energy.

Application in Cancer Care

•	Starving Cancer Cells: The keto diet aims to deprive cancer cells of glucose, potentially making them more vulnerable to conventional treatments like chemotherapy and radiation therapy.

•	Metabolic Effects: Ketogenic metabolism may alter cellular signalling pathways and reduce inflammation, which are factors implicated in cancer progression.

- Weight Management: Some cancer patients benefit from weight loss or weight management support offered by the keto diet, potentially improving overall health outcomes and treatment tolerance.

Potential Benefits

Preclinical research indicates that the ketogenic diet might boost the effectiveness of chemotherapy and radiation therapy by making cancer cells more sensitive to treatment-related stress. This diet restricts carbohydrate intake, leading to lower blood sugar and insulin levels, potentially hindering conditions favourable for cancer cell proliferation. Some individuals undergoing cancer treatment have noted increased energy, clearer thinking, and decreased inflammation while following the ketogenic diet, which can enhance overall well-being.

Considerations

Careful planning is essential for the ketogenic diet to ensure sufficient intake of essential nutrients, vitamins, and minerals. Collaborating with a registered dietitian or healthcare provider is advisable to optimise nutrient balance and address potential deficiencies. The suitability of the keto diet varies among cancer patients, especially those with specific medical conditions, nutritional requirements, or metabolic disorders, necessitating personalised assessment and guidance. Long-term adherence to the keto diet can present challenges due to dietary restrictions and lifestyle adjustments. Exploring flexible approaches or intermittent implementation may be viable options to consider.

The keto diet represents an experimental approach in cancer care, exploring its metabolic effects, potential synergies with conventional treatments, and impact on patient outcomes. Ongoing research aims to elucidate its mechanisms, optimise dietary protocols, and evaluate its safety and efficacy across different cancer types and patient populations.

The ketogenic diet offers promise as an experimental strategy in cancer care, leveraging metabolic changes and potential synergies with conventional treatments to enhance therapeutic outcomes. As research continues to advance, understanding the role of the keto diet in cancer metabolism, treatment response, and patient well-being evolves.

41. Mushroom Extracts: Such as Reishi and Cordyceps for Immune Support

Mushroom extracts, including varieties like Reishi (Ganoderma lucidum) and Cordyceps (Cordyceps sinensis), have been studied for their potential immune-modulating properties and their role in supporting overall health, including in cancer care.

Understanding Mushroom Extracts

•   Traditional Use: Mushrooms like Reishi and Cordyceps have a long history of use in traditional medicine systems, particularly in Asian cultures, for their purported health benefits, including immune support and vitality.

•   Bioactive Compounds: Mushroom extracts contain bioactive compounds such as polysaccharides, beta-glucans, triterpenes, and antioxidants, which contribute to their potential therapeutic effects.

Mushroom extracts are thought to enhance immune function by boosting the activity of immune cells like natural killer (NK) cells and macrophages, which are crucial in identifying and eliminating cancer cells. These extracts also possess antioxidant properties that could potentially reduce oxidative stress and inflammation, promoting overall health and resilience during cancer treatment. As part of integrative cancer care, mushroom extracts are frequently employed to support immune function, improve quality of life, and alleviate side effects associated with treatment.

Potential Benefits

•	Immune Support: Preclinical and clinical studies suggest that mushroom extracts, particularly Reishi and Cordyceps, may strengthen immune responses, improving the body's ability to defend against infections and possibly cancer cells.

•	Anti-inflammatory Effects: Some mushroom extracts exhibit anti-inflammatory properties, which may help alleviate inflammation associated with cancer and its treatment.

•	Quality of Life: Patients using mushroom extracts may experience improved energy levels, reduced fatigue, and enhanced well-being, contributing to better quality of life during cancer treatment.

Considerations

Various mushroom species and their formulations, including extracts, powders, and teas, differ in their levels of bioactive compounds and potential effects. Selecting products from trustworthy sources guarantees reliability and efficacy. Mushroom extracts are generally safe when used according to guidelines, but it's essential to be mindful of potential allergic reactions or interactions with medications. Consulting healthcare providers is advisable, particularly for patients with compromised immune systems. These extracts are commonly used alongside traditional cancer treatments like chemotherapy and radiation therapy as complementary therapies. Collaboration with oncologists and healthcare teams ensures holistic patient care and treatment coordination.

Mushroom extracts represent an experimental approach in cancer care, exploring their immune-modulating effects, antioxidant properties, and potential synergies with conventional treatments. Ongoing research continues to investigate their mechanisms of action, optimal dosing, and impact on treatment outcomes.

Mushroom extracts, such as Reishi and Cordyceps, offer potential benefits in cancer care through their immune-supporting and antioxidant properties. As an experimental therapy, their integration into comprehensive cancer treatment plans under medical guidance allows patients to explore innovative approaches to enhance treatment efficacy, improve quality of life, and support overall well-being.

42. High-Dose Vitamin C: Intravenous Vitamin C Therapy

High-dose vitamin C therapy, particularly administered intravenously (IV), has been explored in cancer care for its potential antioxidant effects, immune-modulating properties, and supportive role alongside conventional treatments.

Vitamin C acts as a powerful antioxidant, combating free radicals that can damage cells and potentially lead to cancer. At higher doses, it boosts immune function by increasing the activity of white blood cells and stimulating the production of antibodies and cytokines essential for immune response. Research indicates that elevated levels of vitamin C might selectively affect cancer cells, potentially triggering apoptosis (cell death) and inhibiting tumour growth in experimental settings. High-dose vitamin C is used as a complementary therapy alongside chemotherapy, radiation therapy, and other standard treatments to enhance their effectiveness and alleviate associated side effects. IV vitamin C therapy may help reduce oxidative stress and inflammation linked to cancer treatments, potentially improving patient tolerance to therapy. Studies show promising interactions between high-dose vitamin C and conventional treatments, potentially improving treatment outcomes and overall patient wellness.

Potential Benefits

IV vitamin C therapy has shown potential in reducing chemotherapy-related toxicity and enhancing quality of life by alleviating side effects like fatigue, nausea, and neuropathy. By bolstering immune function, high-dose vitamin C may aid in fighting infections and maintaining overall immune health throughout cancer treatment. Patients often describe increased energy levels, improved mental clarity, and enhanced well-being during and after IV vitamin C sessions, thereby contributing to an improved overall quality of life.

Considerations

High-dose vitamin C therapy should always be administered under medical supervision to monitor for potential side effects, including kidney stones (particularly in patients with a history of kidney disease) and gastrointestinal discomfort. Treatment protocols for high-dose vitamin C therapy are tailored to individual patient health status, cancer type, treatment stage, and overall treatment objectives. Collaborating closely with healthcare providers ensures the safe and effective integration of IV vitamin C therapy with conventional cancer treatments, maximising therapeutic benefits and improving patient outcomes.

High-dose vitamin C therapy represents an experimental approach in cancer care, exploring its antioxidant effects, immune-modulating properties, and potential synergies with conventional treatments. Ongoing research continues to investigate optimal dosing regimens, safety profiles, and specific mechanisms of action in different cancer types.

High-dose vitamin C therapy offers promise as part of integrative cancer care, leveraging antioxidant benefits, immune support, and potential synergies with conventional treatments. As research advances, understanding the role of IV vitamin C therapy in cancer treatment and patient outcomes evolves.

43. Gerson Therapy: Diet and Detoxification Regimen

Gerson Therapy is a nutritional and detoxification regimen developed by Dr. Max Gerson in the 1920s, focusing on intensive dietary interventions and detoxification to support the body's natural healing processes.

Gerson Therapy promotes a plant-based diet centered around organic fruits, vegetables, and whole grains. Freshly extracted juices, particularly from raw produce, play a vital role in daily nutrition. The therapy also incorporates regular consumption of fresh juices and specialised treatments like coffee enemas to aid liver function and facilitate detoxification. Additionally, it includes nutritional supplements such as potassium, iodine, and pancreatic enzymes to address specific deficiencies and support metabolic functions.

Gerson Therapy aims to provide essential nutrients, antioxidants, and enzymes vital for cellular repair, immune support, and overall well-being during cancer treatment. Advocates argue that it assists in detoxifying the body by eliminating toxins and metabolic waste, thereby reducing oxidative stress and enhancing the body's natural healing abilities. Emphasizing a holistic approach to cancer care, Gerson Therapy focuses on dietary adjustments, detoxification methods, and lifestyle changes to improve treatment effectiveness. A diet rich in fresh fruits and vegetables provides ample vitamins, minerals, and phytochemicals that support immune function and cellular health. In Gerson Therapy, fresh juices and plant-based foods are abundant sources of antioxidants, believed to protect cells from oxidative stress associated with cancer progression. Some individuals have reported increased energy levels, reduced symptoms such as nausea and fatigue, and an overall improvement in well-being while following Gerson Therapy principles.

Considerations

Gerson Therapy should be overseen by medical professionals, particularly for cancer patients actively undergoing treatment or with specific medical conditions affecting dietary tolerance. The therapy involves rigorous adherence to dietary rules, juicing protocols, and detoxification methods, which can be challenging for some patients in terms of adherence and long-term feasibility. Working closely with healthcare providers ensures the safe integration of Gerson Therapy alongside conventional cancer treatments, maximising treatment effectiveness and patient outcomes.

Gerson Therapy represents an experimental approach in cancer care, exploring its nutritional benefits, detoxification effects, and potential synergies with conventional treatments. Ongoing research and anecdotal evidence continue to inform its application and effectiveness in supporting cancer patients' overall health and treatment journey.

Gerson Therapy offers a holistic approach to cancer management, emphasising dietary modifications, detoxification, and nutritional support to complement conventional treatments. As research and clinical experience evolve, understanding the role of Gerson Therapy in cancer care continues to expand.

44. Ozone Therapy: Introducing Ozone to the Body

Ozone therapy involves the introduction of ozone (a molecule consisting of three oxygen atoms) into the body, typically through various methods such as ozone gas, ozone-infused water, or ozonated oils. This therapy is controversial and not widely accepted in mainstream medicine for cancer treatment.

Ozone therapy is believed to affect cells and tissues by inducing oxidative stress, which might influence immune responses and enhance oxygen utilization in the body. This therapy can be administered through various methods: directly injected into the bloodstream or muscle tissue (known as autohemotherapy), consumed as ozonated water to potentially improve oxygen delivery and detoxification, or applied topically as ozonated oils for skin conditions or rectally for gastrointestinal issues. Supporters of ozone therapy suggest it could strengthen immune function, improve circulation, and possess antimicrobial properties, theoretically aiding the body's ability to combat cancer cells. Advocates argue that ozone therapy stimulates the immune system, potentially enhancing its ability to detect and respond to cancer cells. Occasionally used alongside traditional cancer treatments, ozone therapy aims to enhance overall well-being, boost energy levels, and alleviate treatment side effects. However, the inclusion of ozone therapy in cancer care remains controversial due to insufficient robust clinical evidence supporting its effectiveness and concerns about safety, particularly regarding potential oxidative damage to healthy tissues.

Ozone therapy involves risks, including the potential for oxidative stress and tissue damage if administered incorrectly or at high concentrations, underscoring the importance of strict safety protocols and practitioner expertise. Its regulatory status differs across countries and regions, often classified as an experimental or alternative therapy without broad endorsement from mainstream medical organisations. Given its controversial nature and varying acceptance among healthcare providers, informed consent and comprehensive patient education are crucial aspects for those considering ozone therapy.

Ozone therapy represents an experimental approach in cancer care, exploring its potential immunomodulatory effects, oxidative mechanisms, and controversial status in mainstream medical practice. Research continues to investigate its safety, efficacy, optimal dosing protocols, and potential benefits in specific cancer types and patient populations.

Ozone therapy remains a contentious topic in cancer treatment, with proponents advocating its potential benefits in supporting immune function and overall health. However, its use in clinical practice is limited by safety concerns, lack of widespread acceptance, and insufficient clinical evidence. By integrating ozone therapy cautiously into comprehensive cancer treatment plans under expert supervision and in conjunction with conventional therapies, patients and healthcare providers navigate the complexities of experimental approaches while prioritising patient safety and well-being.

45. Laetrile: Extracted from Apricot Seeds

Laetrile, also known as amygdalin or Vitamin B17, is a controversial substance extracted from the seeds of apricots and other fruits. It has been promoted as an alternative cancer treatment, although it lacks scientific support and is not widely accepted in mainstream medicine.

Laetrile, primarily derived from amygdalin found in the seeds and pits of fruits like apricots, almonds, and peaches, is purported to release cyanide when metabolised, which advocates claim can selectively destroy cancer cells. It gained popularity in the 1970s as a natural cancer treatment option promoted as non-toxic compared to chemotherapy, with potential anti-cancer effects. However, its efficacy and safety have sparked considerable debate. Regulatory agencies like the FDA have not approved Laetrile for cancer treatment due to insufficient clinical evidence and concerns regarding potential toxicity.

Advocates propose that Laetrile targets cancer cells by releasing cyanide upon metabolism, which is believed to hinder cellular respiration and induce cancer cell death while sparing healthy tissues. However, clinical studies investigating Laetrile's effectiveness have yielded inconclusive results or shown no significant benefits in cancer treatment. The compound's mechanism of action and safety profile remain poorly understood and subject to controversy. Given these uncertainties and potential risks, the use of Laetrile in cancer therapy requires careful consideration and informed decision-making: Cyanide toxicity is a significant concern associated with Laetrile, particularly if not administered under strict medical supervision and in controlled doses. Laetrile lacks approval for cancer treatment in many countries and is deemed an unproven therapy by mainstream medical organisations.

Laetrile represents an experimental approach in cancer care, explored by some patients seeking alternative treatments outside conventional medical practices. Advocates continue to promote its potential benefits, while critics emphasise the lack of scientific validation and the potential risks of cyanide poisoning.

Laetrile remains a controversial and unproven therapy for cancer treatment, lacking robust clinical evidence to support its efficacy and safety. Patients considering Laetrile should engage in thorough research, consult with healthcare providers, and prioritise evidence-based treatments supported by clinical trials and regulatory approval.

Illegal or Dangerous Approaches (Not Recommended)

46. Black Salve: A Corrosive Herbal Paste

Black Salve is a controversial topical paste made from various herbal ingredients, including bloodroot (Sanguinaria canadensis) and zinc chloride. It has been marketed as an alternative treatment for skin cancers and other skin conditions, but it is considered illegal and dangerous by health authorities due to its corrosive nature and lack of scientific evidence supporting its efficacy.

Black Salve typically consists of herbal extracts such as bloodroot, combined with zinc chloride and other ingredients. This topical treatment is directly applied to the skin over suspected cancerous lesions. Advocates claim that Black Salve selectively targets cancer cells, causing necrosis (cell death) and forming an eschar (dead tissue) that eventually sloughs off, supposedly eliminating cancerous tissue. However, regulatory bodies like the FDA have not approved Black Salve for treating cancer or any medical condition. Its use is widely considered illegal and potentially hazardous due to serious safety concerns. There is insufficient clinical research validating the effectiveness and safety of Black Salve. The mechanism by which it purportedly eliminates cancerous tissue lacks robust scientific validation. Black Salve is highly corrosive and poses significant risks to both cancerous and healthy tissues. Its application can lead to severe scarring, infection, and delays in receiving appropriate medical treatment, potentially worsening the patient's condition. Many countries prohibit the sale and promotion of Black Salve for cancer treatment due to its potential dangers and lack of proven therapeutic benefits.

Considerations

•	Patient Safety: The use of Black Salve poses serious risks to patient safety, including tissue damage, infection, and delayed medical intervention. Patients should avoid using Black Salve and seek evidence-based medical treatments.

•	Ethical Concerns: Healthcare providers and regulatory authorities strongly discourage the use of Black Salve due to its potential harm, lack of scientific validation, and exploitation of vulnerable patients seeking alternative cancer treatments.

Black Salve is an illegal and dangerous approach for treating cancer, characterised by its corrosive nature, lack of scientific evidence, and significant health risks. Patients diagnosed with cancer should prioritise evidence-based medical treatments under the guidance of qualified healthcare professionals.

47. Cesium Chloride: Unapproved Mineral Supplement

Cesium Chloride is a controversial mineral supplement that has been promoted as an alternative treatment for cancer, despite lacking approval from regulatory authorities and scientific evidence supporting its efficacy.

Understanding Cesium Chloride

Composition: Cesium Chloride is a salt-like compound composed of cesium, a naturally occurring alkaline metal, combined with chlorine. It is typically marketed in oral supplement form or administered intravenously.

Purported Mechanism: Advocates of Cesium Chloride claim that it raises the pH (alkalinity) of cancer cells, creating an environment that is inhospitable for cancer growth. They suggest that cancer cells cannot survive in alkaline conditions, leading to their destruction.

Controversial Status: Cesium Chloride is not approved for cancer treatment by regulatory agencies like the FDA. Its use is considered controversial due to safety concerns, lack of scientific validation, and potential risks.

Clinical research exploring the effectiveness of Cesium Chloride in cancer treatment is sparse and inconclusive. The proposed mechanisms and therapeutic advantages lack strong scientific evidence. Cesium Chloride has the potential to disturb electrolyte levels, which may result in severe side effects such as cardiac arrhythmias, kidney impairment, and neurological issues. These risks emphasise the necessity for careful management and medical oversight. Marketing and advocating Cesium Chloride as a treatment for cancer are prohibited in numerous jurisdictions due to its lack of approval and potential risks to patients.

Considerations

The utilisation of Cesium Chloride presents substantial risks to patient safety, including the possibility of toxicity and adverse impacts on vital organ functions. It is advisable for patients to refrain from using Cesium Chloride and instead pursue evidence-based medical treatments guided by qualified healthcare professionals. Both healthcare providers and regulatory bodies strongly discourage the use of Cesium Chloride in cancer treatment due to its lack of established effectiveness, potential for harm, and the exploitation of vulnerable patients seeking alternative therapies.

Cesium Chloride is an unapproved and potentially dangerous approach for treating cancer, characterised by its controversial status, lack of scientific evidence, and significant health risks.

48. Urine Therapy: Drinking One's Urine

Urine Therapy, also known as urotherapy or auto-urine therapy, involves the ingestion or application of one's own urine as a supposed remedy for various health conditions, including cancer. This practice is widely regarded as dangerous, ineffective, and lacking scientific validation.

Urine has been historically employed in traditional medicine and various alternative health practices worldwide. Advocates of Urine Therapy assert that urine harbours beneficial substances believed to enhance health and facilitate healing. They propose that urine contains antibodies, hormones, and other bioactive compounds that might potentially bolster the immune system, detoxify the body, and combat cancer cells. However, despite its historical use and anecdotal support, Urine Therapy lacks scientific validation and is not endorsed by mainstream medical authorities for treating cancer or any other medical condition.

Clinical studies exploring the effectiveness of Urine Therapy in cancer treatment are either absent or inconclusive. The idea that consuming urine can cure cancer lacks credible scientific backing. Drinking urine reintroduces harmful substances and potential pathogens into the body, which could result in infections, electrolyte imbalances, and other severe health issues. There is no scientific evidence supporting its efficacy in treating cancer. Urine is expelled from the body as waste for a reason and consuming it does not offer any proven benefits for cancer treatment. This practice can compromise hygiene and overall health, especially problematic for cancer patients who may already have compromised immune systems.

Considerations

Engaging in Urine Therapy presents substantial risks to patient safety, such as possible infections, electrolyte imbalances, and psychological challenges. Patients are advised against using Urine Therapy and encouraged to pursue evidence-based medical treatments under the guidance of qualified healthcare professionals. Healthcare providers and regulatory bodies strongly advise against using Urine Therapy for cancer treatment due to its lack of scientific substantiation, potential risks, and the exploitation of vulnerable patients seeking alternative therapies.

Urine Therapy is an unsafe and ineffective approach for treating cancer, characterised by its controversial status, lack of scientific evidence, and significant health risks.

49. Raw Food Diet: Extreme Dietary Changes Without Medical Supervision

A Raw Food Diet involves consuming predominantly uncooked, unprocessed, and often organic foods such as fruits, vegetables, nuts, seeds, and sprouted grains. Advocates of this diet believe that cooking destroys essential nutrients and enzymes in food, which they claim are necessary for optimal health and potentially beneficial in cancer treatment. However, adopting a Raw Food Diet for cancer treatment is considered dangerous and not recommended without medical supervision.

A Raw Food Diet primarily comprises raw fruits, vegetables, nuts, seeds, and sprouted grains, omitting processed foods, dairy, and most animal products to maintain nutrients and enzymes. Advocates suggest that it can bolster immune function, optimise nutrient absorption, aid detoxification, and potentially hinder cancer cells by reducing processed sugars and fats. Despite its appeal to health-conscious individuals, relying on the Raw Food Diet as a primary cancer treatment lacks scientific backing and may entail substantial health hazards.

Clinical research on the effectiveness of a Raw Food Diet for treating cancer is sparse and inconclusive. Scientific validation of its impact on cancer progression and patient outcomes remains limited. Adopting a Raw Food Diet may result in deficiencies of essential nutrients such as protein, calcium, vitamin B12, iron, and omega-3 fatty acids. These deficiencies can weaken immune function and overall health, which is especially concerning for cancer patients undergoing treatment. Digestive issues and challenges in nutrient absorption from raw foods may further exacerbate nutritional deficiencies, affecting overall well-being negatively.

Considerations

Cancer patients are advised against making drastic dietary changes such as adopting a Raw Food Diet without consulting healthcare professionals. Maintaining proper nutrition during cancer treatment is vital to support immune function, sustain energy levels, and aid in recovery. Any dietary adjustments during cancer treatment should be overseen by qualified healthcare providers who can evaluate nutritional requirements, monitor potential side effects, and offer personalised dietary guidance.

The Raw Food Diet, while emphasising natural, unprocessed foods, is not recommended as a standalone treatment for cancer due to its lack of scientific evidence, potential nutritional deficiencies, and risks to patient health.

50. Injecting Snake Venom: Dangerous and Unproven

Injecting Snake Venom, also known as snake venom therapy or snake venom injections, involves the use of venom extracted from snakes as a purported treatment for various health conditions, including cancer. This practice is highly dangerous, illegal in many jurisdictions, and lacks scientific evidence to support its efficacy.

Snake venom consists of a diverse array of proteins and peptides that exert potent effects on the body, such as neurotoxicity, hemotoxicity, and cytotoxicity. Advocates propose that certain components within snake venom possess anticancer properties. They assert that injecting snake venom can selectively eradicate cancer cells while preserving healthy tissue, potentially inducing apoptosis (cell death) in cancer cells or impeding tumour growth. However, injecting snake venom for cancer treatment lacks approval from regulatory bodies like the FDA and is regarded as an unlawful and potentially perilous practice.

Clinical research examining the effectiveness and safety of injecting snake venom for cancer treatment is either absent or inadequate. The proposed mechanism by which snake venom might combat cancer has not been substantiated through rigorous scientific inquiry. Snake venom is highly toxic and carries substantial risks, including severe allergic reactions, tissue damage, organ failure, and fatalities. These potential adverse effects outweigh any purported benefits suggested by advocates. The sale or endorsement of injecting snake venom as a cancer treatment is prohibited in numerous countries due to the significant dangers associated with its use and the absence of regulatory approval.

Considerations

Injecting snake venom presents immediate and severe risks to patient safety, including systemic toxicity, allergic reactions, and life-threatening complications. Patients are strongly advised against this hazardous practice and should opt for evidence-based medical treatments under the supervision of qualified healthcare professionals. Healthcare providers and regulatory authorities strongly discourage the use of injecting snake venom for cancer treatment due to its lack of scientific validation, potential for harm, and the exploitation of vulnerable patients seeking alternative therapies.

Injecting Snake Venom is an illegal, dangerous, and unproven approach for treating cancer, characterised by its toxicity, lack of scientific evidence, and significant health risks.

Traditional and Cultural Practices

51. Ayurveda: Traditional Indian Medicine

Ayurveda, originating from ancient India, is a holistic system of medicine that has been practiced for thousands of years. It emphasises a personalised approach to health and well-being, balancing the body, mind, and spirit through diet, lifestyle practices, herbal remedies, and therapies. While Ayurveda offers a comprehensive framework for maintaining health and treating various ailments, including cancer, its role in cancer care remains a topic of debate and scrutiny.

Ayurveda is founded on the principle that health and illness stem from the equilibrium or imbalance of three doshas (bio energies): Vata (air and space), Pitta (fire and water), and Kapha (earth and water). Treatment in Ayurveda focuses on reinstating balance through personalised dietary recommendations, lifestyle adjustments, herbal remedies, detoxification therapies, and mind-body practices like yoga and meditation. Ayurvedic practitioners employ various herbs and formulations such as rasayana and chyawanprash, believed to possess therapeutic properties that support overall well-being and potentially alleviate symptoms related to cancer. Prevention through healthy living and customised treatment plans tailored to individual constitutions (prakriti) and imbalances (vikriti) are fundamental principles of Ayurveda.

In the realm of cancer treatment, Ayurveda is frequently employed as a complementary approach aimed at alleviating symptoms, enhancing quality of life, and supporting conventional therapies like surgery, chemotherapy, and radiation. Advocates of Ayurveda propose that specific herbs and treatments can potentially mitigate the side effects of cancer therapies, boost immune function, alleviate inflammation, and promote overall wellness. Examples include turmeric (Curcuma longa), ashwagandha (Withania somnifera), and guduchi (Tinospora cordifolia). Despite widespread use in India and globally, scientific evidence substantiating Ayurveda's efficacy in cancer treatment remains limited and primarily anecdotal. Rigorous clinical trials are essential to validate its safety and effectiveness as part of comprehensive cancer care.

Considerations

Integrating Ayurveda into conventional oncology necessitates close collaboration between Ayurvedic practitioners and oncologists to coordinate care effectively, minimise potential interactions with standard treatments, and enhance patient outcomes. Individuals contemplating Ayurvedic approaches for cancer treatment should consult with experienced Ayurvedic practitioners knowledgeable in oncology. It is crucial to maintain open communication with healthcare providers about all therapies being considered to facilitate comprehensive and safe treatment planning.

Ayurveda offers a holistic approach to health and well-being, encompassing personalised dietary and lifestyle practices, herbal remedies, and therapies rooted in ancient Indian traditions. While Ayurveda may provide supportive care and symptom management for cancer patients, its role in cancer treatment remains adjunctive and should be approached with caution and under the supervision of qualified healthcare professionals.

52. Native American Healing: Ceremonial Practices

Native American Healing encompasses a rich tapestry of traditional practices, ceremonies, and holistic approaches to health and well-being. Rooted in indigenous wisdom and cultural heritage, these healing traditions emphasise spiritual connection, community support, and harmony with the natural world. While specific practices vary among tribes and regions, the overarching principles focus on restoring balance and promoting wellness.

Native American Healing is deeply rooted in spirituality, incorporating ceremonies, rituals, prayers, and connections with ancestral spirits and the natural world. Tribal elders, healers, and shamans, who possess sacred knowledge passed down through generations, guide these healing practices. Ceremonies hold significant importance in Native American Healing, serving as sacred rituals aimed at fostering physical, emotional, and spiritual well-being. Examples include sweat lodge ceremonies, vision quests, drumming circles, smudging (the burning of herbs for cleansing), and healing dances. Healing within Native American traditions emphasises the interconnectedness of mind, body, spirit, and environment, with practices focused on restoring harmony and balance within individuals and their communities.

Native American Healing offers spiritual guidance and solace to cancer patients through ceremonies and rituals designed to cultivate inner strength, resilience, and peace of mind amidst adversity. These healing practices not only provide spiritual support but also foster community solidarity, creating a sense of belonging and shared healing experiences among cancer patients and their families. By honouring ancestral wisdom and traditional values, Native American Healing reinforces cultural identity, resilience, and empowerment among individuals navigating cancer diagnosis and treatment, promoting overall well-being.

It's crucial to honour tribal traditions, customs, and protocols when participating in Native American Healing practices. Cancer patients are encouraged to seek guidance and support from tribal elders, healers, or cultural advisors who deeply appreciate the significance of ceremonies and their healing effects. These practices complement conventional cancer treatments by addressing spiritual and emotional needs, thereby improving quality of life and supporting overall well-being.

Native American Healing embodies centuries-old traditions rooted in spirituality, community, and reverence for the natural world. While its specific impact on cancer treatment outcomes lacks empirical validation, the cultural and spiritual support provided through ceremonies and healing practices can profoundly benefit cancer patients.

53. African Traditional Medicine: Herbal and Spiritual Practices

African Traditional Medicine (ATM) encompasses a diverse array of healing practices, herbal remedies, and spiritual rituals deeply rooted in the continent's rich cultural heritage. For centuries, African communities have relied on traditional healers, known as herbalists, diviners, or shamans, who possess specialised knowledge passed down through oral traditions. ATM integrates holistic principles of health, emphasising harmony between the individual, community, and the natural environment

A cornerstone of African Traditional Medicine (ATM) is the utilisation of medicinal plants and herbal preparations to address various ailments, including cancer. Herbalists play a pivotal role in collecting, preparing, and administering plant-based remedies believed to possess therapeutic properties that facilitate healing and restore bodily balance. Spiritual beliefs and rituals are integral to ATM, acknowledging the interconnectedness of physical health with spiritual and ancestral realms. Healing ceremonies, prayers, and rituals are conducted to seek divine guidance, cleanse negative energies, and reinstate spiritual harmony. ATM underscores the holistic well-being of individuals within their cultural and social frameworks, addressing physical, mental, emotional, and spiritual dimensions of health.

African Traditional Medicine offers diverse herbal remedies believed to aid in cancer treatment by easing symptoms, enhancing immune function, and possibly impeding tumour progression. Examples include extracts derived from plants such as Sutherlandia frutescens (commonly known as cancer bush) and Hypoxis hemerocallidea (African potato). Healing rituals and ceremonies within ATM play a vital role in providing emotional and spiritual support to cancer patients, fostering resilience, optimism, and a sense of community and ancestral connection. ATM reinforces cultural identity, resilience, and empowerment among individuals navigating cancer diagnosis and treatment, honouring ancestral wisdom and enduring practices that have sustained African communities across generations.

Integrating African Traditional Medicine (ATM) into conventional cancer care necessitates close collaboration between traditional healers and healthcare professionals. Effective communication, mutual respect, and coordinated treatment planning are vital to prioritize patient safety and maximise treatment effectiveness. Despite the widespread practice and cultural significance of ATM within African communities, scientific validation of its efficacy in cancer treatment remains limited. Rigorous clinical trials are essential to evaluate the safety, efficacy, and potential interactions of ATM with standard cancer therapies.

African Traditional Medicine embodies a holistic approach to health and healing, integrating herbal remedies, spiritual practices, and cultural resilience. While its specific impact on cancer treatment outcomes requires further scientific investigation, ATM provides valuable support to cancer patients through herbal therapies, spiritual healing, and community solidarity.

54. Shamanic Healing: Using Spiritual Rituals for Healing

Shamanic Healing is a profound spiritual practice found in various indigenous cultures worldwide, rooted in the belief that illness, including cancer, can stem from spiritual disharmony or imbalance. Shamans, spiritual practitioners with unique healing abilities, serve as intermediaries between the human and spirit worlds. Through rituals, ceremonies, and journeys into altered states of consciousness, shamans seek to restore harmony, remove spiritual blockages, and facilitate healing on physical, emotional, and spiritual levels.

Spiritual Intermediaries: Shamans are revered for their ability to communicate with spirits, ancestors, and divine forces to gain insights into the causes of illness and guide healing processes. They often undergo rigorous training and initiation rites to develop their healing abilities.

Rituals and Ceremonies: Shamanic Healing involves a variety of rituals and ceremonies tailored to individual needs, including soul retrieval, energy clearing, purification rituals (such as smudging with sage or other sacred herbs), and spirit journeys (trance-like states induced through drumming, chanting, or dance).

Holistic Approach: Shamanic Healing views health as a state of harmony between the individual, community, and the natural world. It addresses physical ailments by addressing underlying spiritual and emotional imbalances.

Shamanic practitioners provide cancer patients with spiritual guidance and emotional support, assisting them in navigating the challenges they face and cultivating inner strength throughout their healing process. Shamanic rituals are designed to cleanse and harmonise the body's energy fields, fostering relaxation, reducing stress, and potentially aiding the body's innate healing mechanisms. This form of healing also strengthens cultural identity, reconnecting individuals with ancestral wisdom and community support, empowering them to confront their cancer diagnosis and treatment with resilience and spiritual resilience.

Integrating Shamanic Healing into conventional cancer care demands effective communication and cooperation between shamanic practitioners and healthcare providers. This collaborative approach ensures cohesive treatment strategies that emphasise patient safety and overall well-being. Cancer patients interested in Shamanic Healing should seek guidance from seasoned practitioners known for their ethical conduct, adherence to cultural norms, and commitment to addressing both physical and emotional aspects of healing.

Shamanic Healing offers a unique approach to cancer care, emphasising spiritual connection, energetic balance, and cultural resilience. While its specific impact on cancer treatment outcomes requires further scientific exploration, Shamanic Healing provides valuable support through spiritual rituals, ceremonies, and profound insights into the interconnectedness of health and spiritual well-being.

Technological and Future Concepts

55. Nanotechnology: Using Nanoparticles for Targeted Drug Delivery

Nanotechnology represents a cutting-edge approach in cancer treatment, leveraging the unique properties of nanoparticles to deliver drugs directly to cancerous cells while minimising damage to healthy tissues. This innovative field holds promise for enhancing the efficacy of cancer therapies and reducing side effects associated with conventional treatments.

Nanoparticles are minute structures, typically ranging from 1 to 100 nanometres in size, crafted to transport therapeutic agents such as chemotherapy drugs, antibodies, or nucleic acids. These particles can be composed of diverse materials, including lipids, polymers, metals, and biological molecules. A key advantage of nanotechnology in cancer treatment lies in its capacity to deliver drugs directly to cancer cells. Tailored nanoparticles can be engineered to recognise and attach to specific molecules or receptors on cancer cells, thereby augmenting drug absorption and effectiveness while reducing exposure to healthy tissues. Additionally, nanotechnology plays a pivotal role in cancer imaging and diagnostics. Nanoparticles can be designed as contrast agents for advanced imaging methods such as magnetic resonance imaging (MRI), computed tomography (CT), and positron emission tomography (PET), facilitating early detection and precise localisation of tumours.

Nanoparticles serve to encapsulate and shield drugs from degradation in the bloodstream, thereby extending their circulation duration and augmenting their concentration at the tumour site via the enhanced permeability and retention (EPR) effect. This targeted approach enables Nanotechnology to minimise systemic exposure to chemotherapy drugs, thereby alleviating common side effects like nausea, hair loss, and immune suppression associated with traditional chemotherapy. Moreover, nanoparticles facilitate the simultaneous delivery of multiple therapeutic agents, such as combining chemotherapy drugs with immunotherapeutic agents or gene therapy, thereby enabling synergistic treatment strategies tailored to the specific profiles of individual cancers.

Challenges and Considerations

Biocompatibility and Safety: Ensuring the biocompatibility and safety of nanoparticles is crucial for clinical translation. Research focuses on minimising potential toxicity, immune responses, and long-term effects associated with nanoparticle accumulation in the body.

Clinical Translation: While Nanotechnology shows promise in preclinical studies and early-phase clinical trials, scaling up and integrating these technologies into routine clinical practice requires rigorous validation through large-scale clinical trials and regulatory approval processes.

Future Prospects

Nanotechnology has the potential to revolutionise personalised cancer treatment by allowing customisation of nanoparticles according to individual genetic profiles, tumour attributes, and treatment responses. Current research is focusing on developing advanced nanomaterials, responsive smart nanoparticles that react to physiological signals, and theragnostic platforms integrating diagnostics and therapy within a single nanoparticle system.

Nanotechnology represents a transformative approach in cancer treatment, revolutionising drug delivery, imaging, and personalised medicine. While challenges remain in terms of safety, scalability, and clinical integration, ongoing research and technological advancements continue to propel Nanotechnology forward as a promising frontier in the fight against cancer.

56. CRISPR Gene Editing: Editing Genes to Correct Mutations

CRISPR (Clustered Regularly Interspaced Short Palindromic Repeats) gene editing technology represents a revolutionary advancement in biomedical research, offering the potential to precisely alter genetic sequences within cells. This technology has transformative implications for cancer treatment by targeting specific mutations implicated in cancer development and progression.

Genetic Engineering Tool: CRISPR-Cas9 is a powerful genetic engineering tool derived from the immune systems of bacteria. It allows scientists to make precise changes to DNA sequences, either by removing, adding, or altering specific genes within living organisms.

Mechanism: CRISPR-Cas9 functions through a guide RNA (gRNA) that directs the Cas9 enzyme to the desired location on the DNA strand. Cas9 then cuts the DNA at the targeted site, enabling researchers to edit genes by inserting new sequences or correcting existing mutations.

Applications: In cancer research and therapy, CRISPR technology can be used to study oncogenes (genes that promote cancer growth), tumour suppressor genes (genes that inhibit cancer development), and mutations associated with drug resistance or metastasis.

CRISPR-Cas9 technology offers promising avenues in cancer research by targeting and disabling oncogenes responsible for driving cancer cell growth and survival. This approach may effectively stall tumour progression or render cancer cells more susceptible to current treatments. In familial cancers linked to inherited genetic mutations, CRISPR holds potential for correcting these mutations, thereby potentially preventing the onset or advancement of cancer. Moreover, CRISPR can enhance the effectiveness of immunotherapy by genetically modifying immune cells like T cells to improve their ability to identify and eliminate cancer cells, countering the immune evasion strategies employed by tumours.

It is crucial to maintain the specificity of CRISPR-Cas9 when targeting genes to prevent unintended mutations elsewhere in the genome, thereby reducing risks and ensuring safety in clinical settings. Ethical considerations surrounding the use of CRISPR in human genome editing include issues of consent, equitable access to emerging therapies, and broader societal implications arising from alterations to germline (inheritable) genes. These factors underscore the importance of thoughtful and responsible application of CRISPR technology in medical research and treatment.

Future Prospects

CRISPR technology opens up personalised cancer treatments customised to individual genetic profiles, paving the way for targeted therapies that enhance treatment effectiveness. Current research is dedicated to optimising CRISPR techniques, creating efficient in vivo gene editing delivery methods, and extending applications to address complex genetic interactions in cancer beyond single-gene mutations.

CRISPR Gene Editing represents a transformative frontier in cancer research and therapy, harnessing precise genome editing capabilities to address genetic underpinnings of cancer. While challenges in safety, efficacy, and ethical considerations persist, CRISPR technology holds promise for advancing personalised medicine, enhancing treatment options, and ultimately improving outcomes for cancer patients. Continued innovation and ethical stewardship are essential to realising the full potential of CRISPR in the fight against cancer.

57. Bioelectric Treatments: Using Electrical Signals to Influence Cell Behaviour

Bioelectric treatments represent an innovative approach in cancer research and therapy, harnessing electrical signals to modulate cellular behaviour, including proliferation, differentiation, and apoptosis (cell death). This emerging field explores the profound impact of bioelectricity on biological processes, offering potential therapeutic strategies for managing cancer.

Cells in the human body communicate through bioelectric signals that regulate crucial functions like tissue development, wound healing, and immune response. Bioelectric treatments seek to leverage these signals to control cellular behaviours involved in cancer growth and progression. Referred to as bioelectronic devices or electroceuticals, these treatments involve applying electrical stimulation through electrodes or implantable devices to regulate cellular activity at specific sites in the body. Electrical signals can impact ion channels, membrane potentials, and intracellular signalling pathways in cancer cells, influencing their metabolism, response to treatments, and ability to proliferate.

Application in Cancer Therapy

Tumour Modulation: Bioelectric treatments can be applied directly to tumours or cancerous tissues to disrupt cellular pathways essential for tumour survival and progression. This approach may complement existing therapies by sensitising tumours to chemotherapy or radiation.

Electrochemotherapy: Combining electrical pulses with chemotherapy drugs enhances drug uptake by cancer cells, improving treatment efficacy while minimising systemic toxicity to healthy tissues.

Neuromodulation: Electrical stimulation of nerves or neural networks associated with cancer-related pain or symptoms offers palliative care benefits, enhancing patient comfort and quality of life.

Research endeavours are centered on unravelling the bioelectric mechanisms that drive cancer progression and determining the most effective parameters for therapeutic electrical stimulation. Early-stage clinical trials are investigating the safety and effectiveness of bioelectric therapies in cancer patients, evaluating metrics such as tumour response rates, survival outcomes, and enhancements in quality of life.

It is crucial to ensure the precise delivery of bioelectric signals to cancerous tissues while minimising effects on healthy cells to prevent unintended side effects or damage. Effective integration of bioelectric treatments with conventional cancer therapies necessitates interdisciplinary collaboration among oncologists, bioengineers, and electrical engineers. This collaboration aims to refine treatment protocols and enhance treatment outcomes comprehensively.

Future Directions

Personalised Medicine: Advancements in bioelectric treatments hold promise for personalised cancer care, tailoring electrical stimulation parameters to individual patient profiles and tumour characteristics.

Technological Innovations: Ongoing research explores novel bioelectronic devices, advanced electrode technologies, and real-time monitoring systems to enhance precision and efficacy in delivering bioelectric therapies.

Bioelectric treatments represent a frontier in cancer therapy, leveraging electrical signals to modulate cellular behaviours and enhance treatment outcomes. While research continues to elucidate mechanisms and optimise clinical applications, bioelectric therapies offer potential synergies with existing cancer treatments, paving the way for innovative approaches in personalised medicine and improving quality of life for cancer patients worldwide.

58. 3D Printed Organs: Future Possibility for Replacing Cancerous Organs

The advent of 3D printing technology has revolutionised medical research and treatment possibilities, including the potential to fabricate custom-made organs and tissues. This innovation holds promise for addressing the complex challenges of organ failure due to cancer or other diseases, offering a futuristic approach to organ replacement and regeneration.

3D bioprinting employs a methodical process of layering biological materials like cells and biomaterials to construct detailed three-dimensional structures that closely resemble natural tissues and organs. A significant benefit of 3D printed organs is their capacity to be tailored precisely to fit the unique anatomy of each patient, thereby lessening the chances of rejection and enhancing outcomes following transplantation. Biomaterials utilised in bioprinting encompass synthetic polymers, natural biomolecules such as collagen and fibrin, and living cells obtained from the patient's tissues or donor origins.

Application in Cancer Treatment

Organ Replacement: For patients with cancerous organs that require surgical removal (e.g., liver, kidney, or breast tissue), 3D bioprinting offers the potential to create functional replacements tailored to individual patient needs.

Drug Testing and Development: 3D printed tissue models provide platforms for testing new cancer therapies and studying disease mechanisms in a controlled laboratory setting, facilitating personalised treatment approaches.

Regenerative Medicine: Beyond organ transplantation, 3D bioprinting supports tissue regeneration and repair, enabling the development of implantable constructs to enhance healing and recovery after cancer surgery or treatment.

Current Research and Challenges

Bioink Development: Optimisation of bioinks (the printable materials) to ensure cell viability, structural integrity, and compatibility with bioprinting processes remains a critical focus of research.

Vascularisation: Efficient vascularisation (formation of blood vessels) within 3D printed tissues remains a challenge, as adequate blood supply is essential for sustaining larger, complex tissue constructs.

Ethical considerations encompass obtaining informed consent from patients before using bio printed organs or tissues, ensuring they comprehend the risks, benefits, and limitations associated with emerging technologies. Regulatory agencies play a crucial role in setting safety and efficacy standards for bio printed organs, striking a balance between fostering innovation and safeguarding patient welfare in clinical settings.

Future Directions

Progress in 3D bioprinting technologies offers potential for personalised cancer treatment by enabling customised organ replacements and reducing dependence on donor organs. Incorporating robotics, artificial intelligence (AI), and advanced imaging enhances the precision and efficiency of bioprinting intricate tissues and organs.

3D Printed Organs represent a transformative frontier in cancer treatment and regenerative medicine, offering innovative solutions for organ replacement, personalised therapy development, and tissue repair. While challenges in bioink development, vascularisation, and regulatory approval persist, ongoing research and technological advancements continue to propel 3D bioprinting toward clinical reality.

59. Robotic Surgery: Precision Surgery with Robotic Assistance

Robotic surgery represents a significant advancement in surgical techniques, combining the precision of robotics with the expertise of surgeons to perform minimally invasive procedures with enhanced accuracy and control. This technology has revolutionised cancer treatment by enabling complex surgeries with reduced trauma, faster recovery times, and improved outcomes for patients.

Robotic surgery systems, exemplified by the da Vinci Surgical System, utilise robotic arms fitted with miniature surgical tools and a high-definition camera. Surgeons operate these instruments remotely from a console, translating their hand movements into precise actions within the patient's body. Unlike traditional open surgery, robotic-assisted procedures involve small incisions through which instruments and a camera are inserted. This minimally invasive approach reduces blood loss, lowers infection rates, and accelerates recovery compared to conventional surgery. High-definition 3D imaging provides surgeons with detailed, magnified views of the surgical site, improving visualisation of delicate tissues and structures. Robotic systems offer greater dexterity and a wider range of motion than human hands, enabling precise manipulation and suturing during intricate procedures.

Application in Cancer Treatment

Complex Oncological Surgeries: Robotic surgery is utilised in various cancer surgeries, including prostatectomy, hysterectomy, colorectal resections, and thoracic procedures. Its precision and minimally invasive nature enable surgeons to remove tumours with greater accuracy while preserving healthy surrounding tissues.

Lymph Node Dissection: In cancers that spread to nearby lymph nodes, robotic systems facilitate meticulous dissection and removal of affected lymph nodes, reducing the risk of cancer recurrence and improving long-term outcomes.

Reconstructive Procedures: Robotic-assisted reconstructive surgeries, such as breast reconstruction following mastectomy, optimise cosmetic outcomes and patient satisfaction through precise tissue alignment and suturing.

Benefits and Advancements

Minimally invasive robotic procedures are linked to reduced surgical complications, shorter hospital stays, and quicker recovery periods for cancer patients, thereby improving postoperative quality of life. Emerging technologies enable remote or telesurgery, allowing surgeons to perform procedures from distant locations using robotic systems. This capability enhances access to specialised surgical expertise and broadens treatment options for patients in remote or underserved areas.

However, initial costs associated with robotic systems and training can be substantial, which may limit access in certain healthcare settings. Integrating robotic surgery into routine oncological practice necessitates investment in infrastructure and ongoing technical support. Mastery of robotic surgery techniques requires specialised training and proficiency to ensure patient safety, minimise operation time, and optimise surgical outcomes.

Future Directions

AI Integration: Integration of artificial intelligence (AI) algorithms with robotic systems promises to enhance surgical planning, decision-making, and intraoperative guidance, further improving precision and patient outcomes.

Expanding Applications: Ongoing research explores novel applications of robotic surgery in emerging fields such as robotic-assisted radiotherapy, image-guided interventions, and personalised surgical approaches based on patient-specific anatomy and tumour characteristics.

Robotic Surgery represents a transformative innovation in cancer treatment, combining advanced technology with surgical expertise to achieve precise, minimally invasive procedures. While challenges in cost, training, and accessibility persist, robotic systems continue to evolve, offering new possibilities for enhancing surgical precision, improving oncological outcomes, and advancing personalised cancer care in the 21st century.

60. Artificial Intelligence: AI for Personalised Treatment Plans

Artificial Intelligence (AI) has emerged as a powerful tool in oncology, revolutionising the landscape of cancer diagnosis, treatment planning, and patient care. By harnessing vast amounts of patient data, AI algorithms can analyse complex patterns, predict outcomes, and personalise treatment strategies tailored to individual patients.

AI systems leverage a variety of datasets, including genomic profiles, imaging scans, electronic health records (EHRs), and real-time patient monitoring data, to perform comprehensive analyses. Machine learning algorithms process these diverse data inputs to identify biomarkers, detect cancerous lesions, and predict disease progression. Utilising this information, AI-driven platforms develop personalized treatment strategies tailored to individual patient characteristics, such as genetic mutations, tumour biology, treatment history, and response patterns. By optimising therapeutic interventions, AI enhances treatment effectiveness and minimises adverse effects. Clinicians benefit from AI algorithms as decision support tools, gaining insights into treatment recommendations, eligibility for clinical trials, and prognostic assessments, thereby facilitating evidence-based decision-making and improving patient outcomes.

AI plays a pivotal role in precision medicine by pinpointing molecular targets and biomarkers specific to cancer subtypes. This capability enables the customisation of therapies, including targeted treatments, immunotherapies, and combinations, tailored to individual patient profiles, thereby enhancing response rates and survival outcomes. AI-driven radiomics analyse medical imaging data such as CT scans and MRIs to extract quantitative features, predict tumour behaviour, and evaluate treatment responses. This improves diagnostic precision, facilitates early detection, and assists in treatment planning.

Additionally, AI accelerates drug discovery by sifting through extensive compound libraries, forecasting drug efficacy, and identifying new therapeutic targets. This speeds up the development of groundbreaking cancer therapies and personalised treatment strategies.

AI significantly improves diagnostic accuracy and clinical decision-making by analysing intricate datasets and identifying subtle patterns that may elude human observers, thereby mitigating diagnostic errors and enhancing treatment efficacy. By automating repetitive tasks and optimising workflow processes, AI algorithms also streamline operations, allocate resources more efficiently, and increase patient throughput, contributing to improved healthcare delivery and reduced costs. Ensuring the security of patient data from unauthorised access, adhering to regulatory standards such as GDPR and HIPAA, and maintaining data integrity are essential considerations in AI-driven healthcare implementations. Addressing algorithmic bias and promoting equitable access to AI technologies across diverse patient populations are critical steps toward reducing healthcare disparities and advancing overall clinical outcomes.

Future Directions

AI-Integrated Healthcare: Integration of AI with wearable devices, telemedicine platforms, and electronic health records (EHRs) facilitates real-time patient monitoring, remote consultations, and proactive disease management strategies.

Predictive Analytics: AI-enabled predictive models forecast disease progression, identify high-risk patients for preventive interventions, and stratify patients based on personalised risk profiles, supporting early intervention and disease prevention efforts.

Artificial Intelligence represents a transformative paradigm in oncology, enabling personalised cancer care through data-driven insights, predictive analytics, and precision treatment planning. While challenges in data governance, algorithm transparency, and ethical considerations persist, AI-driven innovations continue to advance the frontiers of personalised medicine, offering new avenues for improving cancer outcomes and quality of life for patients worldwide.

Unique and Offbeat Ideas

61. **Laughter Therapy: Using Humour to Improve Mood and Health**

Laughter therapy, also known as humour therapy or laughter yoga, harnesses the healing power of laughter to promote emotional well-being, reduce stress, and enhance overall health. This unconventional approach has gained recognition for its therapeutic benefits in alleviating symptoms and improving quality of life for cancer patients and survivors.

Psychological Benefits: Laughter stimulates the release of endorphins, the body's natural feel-good chemicals, which promote a sense of happiness and relaxation. It reduces stress hormones like cortisol and boosts immune function, contributing to a positive psychological state.

Social Connection: Laughter fosters social interaction and strengthens relationships, creating a supportive environment for cancer patients to share experiences, cope with challenges, and cultivate a sense of community.

Mind-Body Connection: The mind-body connection inherent in laughter therapy emphasises the interplay between mental and physical health, promoting holistic well-being and resilience during cancer treatment.

Practical Applications

Laughter Yoga: Laughter yoga combines simulated laughter exercises with deep breathing techniques to induce genuine laughter and cultivate a playful mindset. Participants engage in laughter sessions led by trained facilitators, promoting relaxation and emotional release.

Comedic Therapy: Incorporating humour and light-hearted activities into cancer support groups, therapy sessions, and hospital settings encourages laughter as a coping mechanism and stress-relief strategy.

Physiological Effects

Laughter boosts immune function by increasing antibody production and activating immune cells, which may help the body fight illness and aid in recovery. The endorphins released during laughter serve as natural painkillers, reducing discomfort and providing relief for cancer patients experiencing pain or undergoing treatment.

Evidence and Research

Research suggests that laughter therapy can improve mood, reduce anxiety, and enhance the quality of life for cancer patients undergoing chemotherapy, radiation, or palliative care. Integrating laughter therapy into comprehensive cancer care may alleviate psychological distress, reduce treatment-related side effects, and foster a more positive outlook during the cancer journey.

Collaboration among oncologists, psychologists, and healthcare providers to include laughter therapy in holistic treatment plans enhances patient-centered care, addressing emotional well-being alongside medical interventions. Providing laughter therapy sessions in oncology wards, infusion centres, and survivorship programs offers relaxation, distraction, and emotional support for cancer patients, caregivers, and healthcare professionals.

Laughter therapy exemplifies a unique and offbeat approach to enhancing emotional resilience, promoting social connection, and improving overall quality of life for individuals navigating the complexities of cancer diagnosis and treatment. While not a replacement for conventional medical therapies, laughter therapy complements comprehensive cancer care by fostering a positive mindset, reducing stress, and empowering patients to embrace moments of joy and laughter amidst the challenges of cancer.

62. Pet Therapy: Spending Time with Animals

Pet therapy, also known as animal-assisted therapy or animal-assisted activities, involves interactions between trained animals and individuals to promote emotional, physical, and social well-being. This unconventional approach has shown promise in providing comfort, reducing stress, and enhancing quality of life for cancer patients and survivors.

Interacting with animals, such as dogs, cats, and horses, can evoke positive emotions, reduce feelings of loneliness, and provide a sense of companionship during the cancer journey. Pets offer unconditional love and support, fostering a nurturing environment for emotional healing. Petting animals has been shown to lower cortisol levels, the stress hormone, promoting relaxation and alleviating anxiety. This physiological response enhances mood and improves overall emotional well-being for cancer patients undergoing treatment.

Additionally, pets serve as social catalysts, facilitating interactions and encouraging communication among patients, caregivers, and healthcare providers. Animal-assisted activities create opportunities for meaningful connections and shared experiences in supportive care settings.

Trained therapy animals visit oncology wards, infusion centers, and outpatient clinics to interact with patients and provide emotional support during treatment sessions. These visits bring moments of joy, distraction, and comfort amid medical procedures. Engaging in activities such as grooming, walking, or playing with therapy animals encourages physical movement, stimulates cognitive function, and fosters a sense of purpose and enjoyment for patients recovering from cancer treatment.

Physiological Benefits

Interacting with animals releases endorphins, the brain's natural pain relievers, which can help alleviate discomfort and improve pain management for cancer patients experiencing physical symptoms. Petting animals has been associated with reduced blood pressure and heart rate, supporting cardiovascular health and promoting relaxation during the stressful situations of cancer treatment.

Evidence and Research

Clinical research demonstrates that pet therapy significantly reduces anxiety, enhances mood, and improves overall quality of life among cancer patients, caregivers, and healthcare professionals in supportive care settings. The enduring benefits include increased resilience, enhanced coping mechanisms, and greater emotional fortitude in navigating the emotional and psychological challenges associated with a cancer diagnosis and treatment journey. Collaborative efforts involving oncologists, psychologists, and trained animal handlers are essential to ensure the safe and effective integration of pet therapy into comprehensive cancer care plans. This approach not only enhances patient safety and adherence to treatment but also fosters holistic well-being. By implementing pet-friendly policies in healthcare facilities and survivorship programs, inclusive environments are created that prioritise patient-centered care, emotional support, and positive therapeutic experiences for those affected by cancer.

Pet therapy exemplifies a unique and beneficial approach to enhancing emotional resilience, reducing stress, and promoting overall well-being for cancer patients and survivors. By fostering meaningful connections with animals, pet therapy contributes to a holistic healing process that addresses the emotional, social, and psychological dimensions of the cancer journey. While not a substitute for medical treatment, pet therapy complements conventional therapies by providing comfort, companionship, and therapeutic benefits that support a positive quality of life during and after cancer treatment.

63. Forest Bathing: Immersing Oneself in Nature

Forest bathing, or Shinrin-yoku in Japanese, is a practice that involves immersing oneself in natural surroundings, particularly forests, to enhance physical, mental, and emotional well-being. This therapeutic approach has gained popularity for its ability to reduce stress, boost immune function, and promote relaxation, offering potential benefits for cancer patients and survivors.

Forest bathing harnesses the healing power of nature by engaging all the senses in a peaceful forest environment. Participants immerse themselves in the sights, sounds, smells, and textures of the forest, fostering a deep sensory connection with their natural surroundings. Time spent in nature, away from daily life's hustle and bustle, reduces cortisol levels, lowers blood pressure, and induces relaxation. This physiological response helps alleviate stress, anxiety, and mental fatigue often associated with cancer treatment. Forest bathing encourages mindfulness practices such as deep breathing, meditation, and conscious observation of natural elements. These techniques enhance self-awareness, promote calmness, and support mental clarity and emotional resilience.

Certified forest therapy guides lead participants through structured walks in natural environments, incorporating relaxation exercises, mindfulness activities, and sensory immersion techniques. Individuals can also practice forest bathing independently by selecting serene forest settings, disconnecting from electronic devices, and engaging in leisurely activities such as walking, sitting quietly, or journaling amidst nature. Phytoncides, volatile compounds released by trees and plants, possess antimicrobial properties that enhance immune function and boost natural killer cell activity, potentially aiding in immune system regulation during cancer recovery. Exposure to nature increases serotonin and dopamine levels, neurotransmitters that regulate mood and emotional well-being. Forest bathing promotes a positive outlook, reduces depressive symptoms, and improves overall mental health.

Research studies have demonstrated that forest bathing enhances physiological indicators such as heart rate variability and cortisol levels, indicating reduced stress and increased relaxation responses. These findings highlight the therapeutic benefits of nature-based therapies in promoting overall health and well-being. Regular participation in forest bathing provides lasting benefits such as improved sleep quality, reduced inflammation, and enhanced resilience to stress, all of which contribute to better recovery and quality of life enhancements for cancer patients and survivors. Integrating forest bathing into comprehensive wellness programs and supportive care services allows cancer patients the opportunity to rejuvenate, recharge, and reconnect with natural environments. This inclusion not only complements conventional medical treatments but also addresses emotional and psychosocial needs alongside clinical interventions. To ensure equitable access to nature-based therapies for diverse patient populations affected by cancer, it is crucial to promote inclusive practices and provide accessible natural settings for forest bathing initiatives.

Forest bathing offers a unique and therapeutic approach to enhancing well-being, reducing stress, and fostering resilience among cancer patients and survivors. By immersing oneself in natural environments, individuals can experience profound healing benefits that support physical, emotional, and psychological health throughout the cancer journey. While not a substitute for medical treatment, forest bathing complements conventional therapies by promoting relaxation, boosting immune function, and cultivating a deeper connection with nature, contributing to a holistic approach to cancer care and survivorship.

64. Volunteering: Helping Others to Find Purpose and Joy

Volunteering is a meaningful and altruistic activity that involves dedicating time and effort to support others in need. Engaging in volunteer work not only benefits the recipients but also offers significant rewards for the volunteers themselves, including a sense of purpose, fulfilment, and emotional well-being. For cancer patients and survivors, volunteering provides an opportunity to contribute positively to their communities, find joy in helping others, and enhance their overall quality of life.

Volunteering offers individuals a profound sense of purpose and fulfilment, especially during difficult times like a cancer diagnosis and treatment. It brings a sense of achievement and satisfaction through positively impacting the lives of others. Supporting others can uplift spirits, alleviate feelings of loneliness, and foster a deeper connection with the community. Volunteering encourages social interaction, boosts self-esteem, and bolsters emotional strength throughout the cancer experience. Participating in volunteer work can redirect focus from personal struggles and concerns related to cancer, providing a much-needed respite and lowering stress levels. The act of assisting others releases endorphins and cultivates a positive emotional state.

Practical Ways to Volunteer

Peer Support Programs: Joining peer support groups for cancer patients and survivors allows individuals to share their experiences, offer encouragement, and provide emotional support to others facing similar challenges.

Hospital and Clinic Support: Volunteering at hospitals, oncology centres, or cancer clinics involves assisting patients, caregivers, and healthcare professionals, offering comfort, companionship, and practical assistance during treatment.

Community Outreach: Participating in community outreach events, fundraisers, or awareness campaigns raises awareness about cancer-related issues, advocates for cancer research, and supports community efforts to improve cancer care and support services.

Volunteering offers chances to acquire new skills, explore various roles, and develop both personally and professionally. These experiences can be instrumental for personal growth and future career prospects. Engaging in volunteer work builds new friendships, strengthens social circles, and forges meaningful connections with like-minded individuals who share similar interests and values. Establishing supportive relationships enhances emotional well-being and bolsters social support networks.

Integration into Cancer Care

Incorporating volunteer roles into cancer wellness programs and survivorship initiatives empowers individuals to play an active role in their recovery journey, foster community involvement, and nurture a sense of purpose and belonging. Balancing volunteer responsibilities with self-care routines, medical treatments, and personal well-being ensures that volunteering remains a beneficial and sustainable activity that improves overall quality of life.

Volunteering offers a unique and fulfilling approach to supporting others, finding purpose, and enhancing well-being for cancer patients and survivors. By giving back to the community and helping those in need, individuals affected by cancer can experience meaningful connections, personal growth, and emotional resilience throughout their cancer journey.

65. Traveling: Experiencing New Places for Mental Refreshment

Traveling is a transformative experience that offers mental refreshment, personal growth, and a sense of renewal for individuals affected by cancer. Whether exploring distant destinations or embarking on local adventures, traveling provides opportunities to rejuvenate the mind, reconnect with oneself, and create lasting memories.

Mindful Distraction: Traveling serves as a mindful distraction from cancer-related stressors, treatment routines, and daily challenges. Immersing oneself in new environments stimulates curiosity, promotes relaxation, and encourages a shift in perspective, fostering mental clarity and emotional resilience.

Cultural Exploration: Experiencing different cultures, traditions, and landscapes enriches personal understanding, broadens perspectives, and promotes cultural appreciation. Engaging in local customs, trying new cuisines, and connecting with diverse communities enhances the travel experience and promotes overall well-being.

Emotional Healing: Traveling allows individuals to escape familiar surroundings, embrace spontaneity, and embark on transformative journeys of self-discovery and emotional healing. Exploring natural wonders, historical landmarks, or spiritual retreats provides moments of introspection, inspiration, and inner peace.

Before embarking on a trip, it's advisable to consult healthcare providers to assess your health status, obtain necessary medical clearances, and address specific travel concerns related to cancer treatment, medications, and immune system health. Plan travel itineraries that prioritise medical needs and ensure access to healthcare facilities if necessary. Traveling with trusted companions, such as family members, friends, or support networks, not only enhances safety but also provides emotional support and fosters shared experiences that strengthen relationships and offer mutual encouragement during the journey. Select travel destinations that offer accessibility features, accommodations, and amenities tailored to individual mobility needs, ensuring physical comfort and overall well-being. Factors to consider include wheelchair accessibility, availability of medical facilities, and proximity to supportive resources.

Participating in wellness retreats, spa vacations, or nature-based excursions provides opportunities to relax, rejuvenate, and prioritise self-care in peaceful settings. These retreats support comprehensive healing, offering stress relief and mindfulness practices that enhance both emotional and physical well-being. Traveling to commemorate significant milestones in the cancer journey, such as treatment milestones, remission anniversaries, or personal achievements, allows individuals to recognise progress, cultivate resilience, and cherish moments that affirm life and inspire hope for the future. Incorporating travel into the cancer experience encourages personal growth, self-expression, and adaptive coping strategies that strengthen resilience and empower individuals to face life's challenges with courage and optimism. Travel becomes a form of self-nurturing and empowerment, contributing to overall well-being. Engaging with travel support networks, online communities, or agencies specialising in accessible and inclusive travel facilitates planning, meets specific needs, and ensures safe and enjoyable travel experiences for those affected by cancer.

Traveling offers a transformative and rejuvenating experience that promotes mental refreshment, personal growth, and emotional healing for cancer patients and survivors. By exploring new places, embracing cultural diversity, and celebrating life's milestones, individuals can cultivate resilience, find inspiration, and create meaningful memories that enrich the cancer journey

66. Learning a New Skill: Keeping the Mind Engaged and Active

Learning a new skill is a powerful way for cancer patients and survivors to keep their minds engaged, foster personal growth, and maintain a sense of purpose and accomplishment. Whether exploring creative arts, acquiring practical abilities, or delving into intellectual pursuits, acquiring new skills promotes cognitive stimulation, emotional well-being, and resilience throughout the cancer journey.

Mental Stimulation: Engaging in learning activities stimulates cognitive function, enhances neural connections, and promotes brain health. Learning new skills challenges the mind, improves concentration, and supports mental acuity, which is beneficial for cognitive resilience during and after cancer treatment.

Sense of Achievement: Mastering a new skill fosters a sense of accomplishment, boosts self-esteem, and instils confidence in one's abilities. Celebrating personal achievements, no matter how small, encourages a positive outlook, promotes resilience, and reinforces a sense of purpose beyond cancer diagnosis and treatment.

Emotional Well-being: Learning new skills provides a positive distraction from cancer-related stressors, treatment routines, and emotional challenges. It offers opportunities for creative expression, personal growth, and self-discovery, which contribute to emotional resilience and overall well-being.

Practical Ways to Acquire New Skills

Engaging in artistic pursuits like painting, sculpture, photography, writing, or music provides a creative outlet for emotional expression, fosters creativity, and uncovers hidden talents. Participating in art classes, workshops, or online tutorials offers structured learning environments and encourages artistic exploration. Developing practical skills such as cooking, gardening, woodworking, or home improvement enhances daily life, promotes self-sufficiency, and instils a sense of achievement. Joining community classes, vocational training programs, or hobby groups nurtures skill development within supportive communities. Pursuing intellectual interests like learning a new language, delving into history, exploring scientific concepts, or engaging in philosophical discourse stimulates curiosity, expands knowledge, and hones critical thinking abilities. Online courses, educational materials, and local libraries provide accessible avenues for intellectual enrichment.

Incorporating skill-building activities into cancer care enhances therapeutic engagement, stimulates cognitive function, and fosters adaptive coping mechanisms. Acquiring new skills serves as a pathway to self-care, empowerment, and personal development, contributing positively to overall well-being and quality of life. Establishing supportive environments, such as cancer support groups, wellness programs, or community centres, promotes peer encouragement, shared learning, and mutual inspiration among those affected by cancer. These settings cultivate a sense of community, camaraderie, and emotional support during skill-building pursuits.

Considerations for Cancer Patients and Survivors

Taking into account physical constraints, treatment schedules, and energy levels when choosing educational activities ensures accessibility and encourages comfortable participation. Adaptations like assistive technologies, personalised learning strategies, and flexible scheduling cater to individual requirements and preferences. Balancing learning initiatives with self-care routines, medical appointments, and restorative practices promotes a comprehensive approach to well-being and sustains involvement in skill development. Prioritising health, heeding one's body signals, and consulting healthcare professionals enhance the advantages of learning throughout the cancer experience.

Learning a new skill offers cancer patients and survivors a transformative journey of personal growth, cognitive stimulation, and emotional resilience. By engaging in creative arts, acquiring practical abilities, or pursuing intellectual interests, individuals cultivate self-expression, celebrate achievements, and discover newfound strengths that enrich their lives beyond cancer.

67. Playing Music: Engaging in Musical Activities

Music has the profound ability to uplift spirits, soothe anxieties, and ignite the soul with its harmonies and rhythms. For those navigating the challenging terrain of cancer diagnosis and treatment, engaging in musical activities offers a therapeutic sanctuary—a place where emotions find expression, minds find respite, and spirits find renewal. Whether through the gentle strum of a guitar, the resonance of a piano's keys, or the heartfelt lyrics of a song, music becomes not just a pastime but a healing companion on the journey towards wellness and resilience.

In the realm of cancer care, where the focus often centres on medical treatments and physical well-being, music emerges as a powerful ally in addressing the emotional and psychological aspects of healing. It transcends language barriers, cultural divides, and physical limitations, offering a universal language of comfort and connection. Through playing instruments, singing, or participating in music therapy sessions, individuals affected by cancer discover pathways to emotional release, cognitive stimulation, and personal empowerment.

Playing music is more than a creative pursuit; it is a transformative experience that invites individuals to reclaim their sense of agency amidst the uncertainties of illness. It encourages self-expression, fosters camaraderie with fellow musicians, and provides moments of joy and inspiration in the midst of medical challenges. Whether learning new melodies, revisiting familiar tunes, or improvising harmonies, each musical endeavour becomes a testament to resilience and a celebration of life's enduring rhythms.

68. Gardening: Connecting with Nature and Growing Plants

Amidst the tumultuous journey of battling cancer, finding moments of tranquillity and healing can be as simple as connecting with the earth and nurturing life. Gardening offers a therapeutic oasis where individuals affected by cancer can cultivate hope, resilience, and a profound connection with the natural world. Beyond its role in providing fresh produce or vibrant flowers, gardening becomes a transformative practice—a source of physical activity, emotional solace, and spiritual renewal.

At its core, gardening provides a sanctuary of sensory delights and tangible rewards. The act of planting seeds, tending to seedlings, and witnessing their growth mirrors the journey of resilience in the face of adversity. It offers a tangible reminder that life continues to thrive and renew itself, even amidst the challenges of illness. For cancer patients undergoing treatment, the gentle physical exertion involved in gardening can promote strength, flexibility, and a sense of accomplishment, contributing to overall well-being.

The therapeutic benefits of gardening extend beyond physical activity. Engaging with nature has been scientifically shown to reduce stress levels, lower blood pressure, and elevate mood. The sights, smells, and textures of the garden evoke a sense of peace and serenity, providing a welcome reprieve from the clinical environment of hospitals and treatment centres. As individuals immerse themselves in the rhythms of planting, watering, and nurturing plants, they experience a profound connection with the earth—a connection that nurtures the spirit and replenishes the soul.

Moreover, gardening fosters a sense of purpose and empowerment. It allows individuals to play an active role in their healing journey, fostering a sense of agency and control amidst the uncertainties of illness. Whether cultivating a vegetable patch, designing a flower bed, or simply tending to potted plants on a balcony, each gardening endeavour becomes a testament to resilience, creativity, and the enduring cycle of life.

69. Cooking: Preparing Healthy Meals

Cooking isn't just a chore; it's a creative act of nourishment that can empower cancer patients and survivors on their journey to healing. In the midst of medical treatments and lifestyle adjustments, preparing healthy meals becomes a therapeutic endeavour—a way to nurture the body, engage the senses, and reclaim a sense of control over one's health and well-being.

For cancer patients undergoing treatment, maintaining a nutritious diet is essential for supporting immune function, managing side effects, and promoting overall health. Cooking at home allows individuals to tailor meals to their dietary needs and preferences, ensuring they receive essential nutrients while avoiding processed foods and excessive sugars that can compromise health.

Beyond its nutritional benefits, cooking offers a gateway to sensory pleasure and emotional satisfaction. The aromas of fresh herbs, the vibrant colours of seasonal produce, and the tactile experience of chopping and stirring evoke a sense of mindfulness and engagement with the present moment. This sensory immersion can be particularly therapeutic during times of stress or uncertainty, providing a grounding experience that nurtures the mind and spirit.

Cooking encourages creativity and self-expression. Experimenting with new recipes, exploring diverse cuisines, and incorporating wholesome ingredients can inspire a sense of culinary adventure and discovery. For cancer survivors adjusting to post-treatment life, rediscovering the joy of cooking fosters a sense of empowerment and resilience, reaffirming their ability to make positive choices for their health and well-being.

Cooking promotes social connection and shared experiences. Inviting loved ones to join in meal preparation or hosting gatherings centered around healthy eating creates opportunities for bonding and support. Sharing nourishing meals with family and friends fosters a sense of community and reinforces the importance of holistic care in the journey towards recovery.

Diet and Nutrition

70. Organic Foods: Eating Organic Produce to Avoid Pesticides

In the context of cancer prevention and treatment, dietary choices play a pivotal role in supporting overall health and well-being. Organic foods have gained significant attention not only for their potential nutritional benefits but also for their reduced exposure to synthetic pesticides, herbicides, and genetically modified organisms (GMOs). For cancer patients and survivors, opting for organic produce represents a conscious effort to minimise environmental toxins and support the body's natural defences during treatment and recovery.

Organic farming practices prioritise sustainable methods that exclude the use of synthetic chemicals. Instead, organic farmers rely on natural fertilisers, crop rotation, and biological pest control to maintain soil health and productivity. This approach not only reduces the risk of chemical residues in food but also promotes biodiversity and supports ecosystems that contribute to long-term environmental sustainability.

One of the primary motivations for choosing organic foods is the avoidance of pesticide exposure. Pesticides used in conventional agriculture have been linked to potential health risks, including disruption of hormone function, immune suppression, and carcinogenic effects. By opting for organic fruits, vegetables, and grains, individuals can mitigate these risks and enhance their nutritional intake with produce that is free from potentially harmful residues.

Research suggests that organic foods may offer nutritional advantages as well. Studies have shown that organic produce tends to contain higher levels of certain nutrients and antioxidants compared to conventionally grown counterparts. For instance, organic fruits and vegetables have been found to have higher concentrations of vitamin C, antioxidants like flavonoids, and essential minerals such as iron and magnesium. These nutritional benefits are particularly valuable for cancer patients, who may have increased nutrient needs due to the demands of treatment and recovery.

Furthermore, organic foods support broader principles of sustainable agriculture and environmental stewardship. By supporting organic farming practices, consumers contribute to reducing pollution, conserving water resources, and protecting soil health. Organic agriculture promotes soil biodiversity and resilience, which is crucial for maintaining productive and sustainable food systems in the face of climate change and environmental challenges.

Incorporating organic foods into a cancer-fighting diet involves making informed choices about food sourcing and understanding labelling standards. Look for certified organic labels that indicate compliance with rigorous standards for organic production. While organic foods may sometimes be more expensive or less accessible, prioritising organic options for high-risk foods such as berries, leafy greens, and grains can maximise the health benefits while minimising potential exposure to harmful chemicals.

Choosing organic foods is a proactive step towards supporting overall health and reducing environmental impact. For cancer patients and survivors, the decision to incorporate organic produce into their diet aligns with efforts to optimize nutrition, minimise toxin exposure, and promote sustainable food systems. By embracing organic foods, individuals can cultivate a diet that not only supports their journey towards wellness but also contributes to a healthier planet for future generations.

71. Juicing: Consuming Fresh Vegetable and Fruit Juices

Juicing has gained popularity as a convenient and nutrient-rich way to supplement the diet with essential vitamins, minerals, and antioxidants found in fresh fruits and vegetables. For cancer patients and survivors, juicing offers a concentrated source of nutrients that are easily absorbed by the body, supporting immune function, detoxification, and overall vitality.

Freshly extracted juices provide a plethora of health benefits, particularly when using organic produce. Organic fruits and vegetables are free from synthetic chemicals, making them ideal candidates for juicing to reduce toxin exposure. Juices rich in antioxidants such as vitamins A, C, and E, as well as phytochemicals like flavonoids and carotenoids, can help combat oxidative stress and inflammation—two factors implicated in cancer development and progression.

Moreover, juicing offers a practical solution for individuals who may experience challenges in chewing or digesting whole fruits and vegetables due to cancer treatments or oral health issues. The process of juicing breaks down fibre, making it easier for the body to absorb essential nutrients without taxing the digestive system. This can be particularly beneficial for maintaining adequate nutrient intake during periods of reduced appetite or dietary restrictions.

Juicing also provides versatility in creating personalised blends that cater to specific nutritional needs and taste preferences. For example, incorporating cruciferous vegetables like kale, broccoli, and cabbage into juices can provide sulphur-containing compounds known for their anti-cancer properties. Adding citrus fruits rich in vitamin C or ginger and turmeric for their anti-inflammatory benefits can further enhance the therapeutic potential of juices in supporting overall health and well-being.

While juicing offers numerous health benefits, it is essential to approach it as a complement to a balanced diet rather than a sole source of nutrition. Juices should be consumed in moderation to avoid excessive sugar intake from fruit juices and to maintain a diverse intake of whole foods that provide essential fibre and other nutrients. Additionally, consulting with a healthcare provider or registered dietitian can help tailor juicing practices to individual health needs and ensure compatibility with ongoing cancer treatments.

Juicing organic fruits and vegetables can be a valuable addition to a cancer-fighting diet, offering a convenient and nutrient-rich way to support immune function, detoxification, and overall wellness. By harnessing the power of fresh juices, individuals affected by cancer can nourish their bodies with vital nutrients and antioxidants, promoting resilience and vitality throughout their journey towards healing and recovery.

72. Superfoods: Incorporating Foods like Turmeric, Ginger, and Garlic

In the realm of cancer prevention and management, superfoods have gained recognition for their potent medicinal properties and potential health benefits. These nutrient-dense foods, such as turmeric, ginger, and garlic, are celebrated not only for their culinary versatility but also for their rich content of bioactive compounds that possess antioxidant, anti-inflammatory, and immune-supportive properties.

Turmeric is renowned for its active compound curcumin, which has been extensively studied for its anti-cancer properties. Curcumin exhibits antioxidant effects that help neutralise free radicals, which can damage cells and contribute to cancer development. Additionally, curcumin has shown promise in inhibiting cancer cell growth and proliferation, as well as enhancing the body's ability to combat inflammation—a critical factor in cancer progression.

Ginger is another powerful superfood known for its anti-inflammatory and antioxidant properties. Gingerols, the main bioactive compounds in ginger, have demonstrated anti-cancer effects in various preclinical studies. Gingerols have been shown to induce apoptosis (programmed cell death) in cancer cells and inhibit the formation of new blood vessels that supply tumours, thereby impeding their growth and spread.

Garlic is prised not only for its distinctive flavour but also for its potential health benefits. Garlic contains sulphur compounds such as allicin, which have been linked to anti-cancer effects. These compounds have shown promise in slowing the growth of cancer cells and reducing the risk of certain cancers, particularly those affecting the digestive system. Garlic's immune-boosting properties also support overall health and resilience during cancer treatment.

Incorporating superfoods like turmeric, ginger, and garlic into a cancer-fighting diet can be achieved through various culinary approaches. Adding fresh turmeric or turmeric powder to curries, soups, and smoothies infuses dishes with its vibrant colour and distinct flavour, while providing a potent dose of curcumin. Similarly, incorporating fresh or powdered ginger into teas, stir-fries, and marinades enhances both the taste and nutritional profile of meals, while supporting immune function and reducing inflammation.

Garlic can be incorporated into numerous savoury dishes, such as sauces, dressings, and roasted vegetables, to impart its characteristic flavour and health benefits. Consuming raw garlic is believed to maximise its bioavailability of active compounds, although cooked garlic also retains significant nutritional value. The versatility of these superfoods allows individuals to tailor their incorporation into meals according to personal preferences and dietary needs.

While superfoods offer valuable nutritional benefits, they are most effective when integrated into a balanced and varied diet that includes a diversity of whole foods. Consulting with a healthcare provider or registered dietitian can help individuals optimise their diet to support cancer treatment outcomes and overall well-being. It's important to note that while superfoods can complement cancer treatment efforts, they should not be viewed as a substitute for conventional medical therapies.

73. Probiotics: Supporting Gut Health with Fermented Foods

The role of gut health has gained increasing recognition for its impact on overall immune function, inflammation levels, and even the efficacy of cancer therapies. Probiotics, which are beneficial live bacteria and yeasts, play a crucial role in maintaining a healthy balance of gut microbiota—essential for supporting digestion, immune function, and overall well-being.

Understanding Probiotics:

Probiotics are live microorganisms that, when consumed in adequate amounts, confer health benefits on the host. These beneficial bacteria and yeasts are found naturally in certain fermented foods and dietary supplements. The most common types of probiotics include strains of Lactobacillus and Bifidobacterium, which are known for their ability to support digestive health and immune function.

The gut microbiota plays a crucial role in regulating inflammation and immune responses throughout the body. A diverse and balanced gut microbiome is linked to improved digestion, better absorption of nutrients, and reduced inflammation, all essential for supporting overall health and resilience during cancer treatment and recovery. For cancer patients, maintaining optimal gut health is critical because treatments like chemotherapy and radiation therapy can impact digestive function. Probiotics have demonstrated potential in alleviating treatment-related side effects such as diarrhoea, constipation, and gastrointestinal discomfort. They may also aid in bolstering the immune system, which can be compromised during cancer treatment.

Probiotics naturally occur in various fermented foods, making them readily available as part of a balanced diet. Examples of probiotic-rich foods include yogurt (containing live and active cultures), kefir, sauerkraut, kimchi, miso, and kombucha. These foods undergo fermentation, a process that increases their probiotic content and promotes the growth of beneficial microorganisms. Incorporating probiotic-rich foods into a cancer-fighting diet can be achieved through diverse culinary methods. Adding yogurt or kefir to smoothies, incorporating sauerkraut or kimchi into salads or side dishes, and enjoying miso soup or kombucha as beverages are delicious ways to incorporate probiotics into daily meals.

While probiotics offer numerous health benefits, it's essential to choose products that contain live and active cultures and to consume them regularly to maintain a healthy gut microbiome. Individuals undergoing cancer treatment should consult with their healthcare team before starting probiotic supplements, as specific strains and dosages may be recommended based on individual health needs and treatment protocols.

Incorporating probiotics into a cancer-fighting diet supports gut health, enhances immune function, and may help alleviate digestive issues associated with cancer treatment. By embracing probiotic-rich foods as part of a balanced nutritional approach, individuals affected by cancer can nurture their overall well-being and promote resilience throughout their journey towards healing and recovery.

74. Anti-Inflammatory Diet: Reducing Inflammation Through Diet

Inflammation is a natural immune response crucial for fighting infections and healing wounds. However, chronic inflammation is increasingly recognised as a contributor to the onset and advancement of various diseases, including cancer. An anti-inflammatory diet focuses on consuming foods that lower inflammation levels in the body, supporting overall health and potentially aiding in cancer prevention and treatment. Chronic inflammation can create an environment conducive to cancer by facilitating cancer cell growth, proliferation, and spread. Inflammatory processes can also damage cells, increase oxidative stress, and weaken immune function, all of which are factors in cancer development and progression. Therefore, adopting dietary strategies to mitigate inflammation is considered beneficial for both cancer prevention and management.

An anti-inflammatory diet emphasises whole, nutrient-dense foods that are rich in antioxidants, omega-3 fatty acids, and phytochemicals known for their anti-inflammatory properties. Key components of an anti-inflammatory diet include:

Fruits and Vegetables: Colourful fruits and vegetables are abundant in antioxidants such as vitamins A, C, and E, as well as phytochemicals like flavonoids and carotenoids. These compounds help neutralise free radicals and reduce oxidative stress, which can contribute to inflammation and cancer development.

Healthy Fats: Omega-3 fatty acids found in fatty fish (e.g., salmon, mackerel, sardines), flaxseeds, chia seeds, and walnuts have potent anti-inflammatory effects. These fats help balance the body's inflammatory response and support cardiovascular health.

Whole Grains: Whole grains like oats, quinoa, brown rice, and whole wheat provide fibre and essential nutrients that promote digestive health and contribute to a stable blood sugar level. They also contain phytonutrients that possess anti-inflammatory properties.

Lean Proteins: Lean sources of protein such as poultry, legumes (beans and lentils), and tofu provide essential amino acids without the saturated fats found in red and processed meats, which can contribute to inflammation.

Herbs and Spices: Turmeric, ginger, garlic, cinnamon, and cayenne pepper are examples of herbs and spices known for their anti-inflammatory and antioxidant properties. Incorporating these flavourful additions into meals can enhance the diet's anti-inflammatory benefits.

Benefits of an Anti-Inflammatory Diet in Cancer Care:

For individuals undergoing cancer treatment, managing inflammation is crucial for maintaining overall health and supporting treatment outcomes. An anti-inflammatory diet can help mitigate treatment-related side effects such as fatigue, nausea, and immune suppression. By reducing chronic inflammation, this dietary approach may also enhance the body's ability to heal and recover from cancer therapies.

While an anti-inflammatory diet offers numerous health benefits, it is essential to personalise dietary choices based on individual health needs, preferences, and treatment protocols. Consulting with a registered dietitian or healthcare provider can provide tailored guidance on incorporating anti-inflammatory principles into a cancer-fighting diet.

Adopting an anti-inflammatory diet rich in fruits, vegetables, healthy fats, whole grains, and antioxidant-rich herbs and spices can play a valuable role in reducing inflammation, supporting immune function, and promoting overall well-being during cancer treatment and beyond. By nourishing the body with anti-inflammatory foods, individuals affected by cancer can empower themselves with a proactive approach to enhancing their health and resilience.

Social and Environmental Changes

75. **Building a Support Network: Surrounding Oneself with Supportive People**

Receiving a cancer diagnosis can be profoundly overwhelming and emotionally taxing. Establishing a robust support network is crucial for individuals navigating the complexities of cancer treatment and recovery. This network typically comprises family members, friends, healthcare professionals, and fellow cancer survivors who offer emotional, practical, and sometimes financial assistance throughout the journey. Numerous studies underscore the significant role of social support in enhancing health outcomes and improving quality of life for cancer patients. A strong support system can mitigate feelings of isolation, anxiety, and depression commonly experienced with cancer. It fosters a sense of belonging, provides encouragement, and offers reassurance that one is not confronting the challenges alone.

Types of Supportive Relationships:

Family and Friends: Loved ones play a crucial role in offering emotional support, companionship, and practical assistance. They can provide transportation to medical appointments, help with household chores, or simply lend a listening ear during difficult moments.

Healthcare Team: Building a trusting relationship with healthcare providers—oncologists, nurses, social workers, and counsellors—is vital. These professionals offer medical expertise, treatment guidance, and emotional support tailored to the individual's medical needs and personal preferences.

Peer Support Groups: Connecting with other cancer patients and survivors through support groups or online communities can be incredibly beneficial. Peer support provides a unique opportunity to share experiences, exchange information, and gain insights from those who understand firsthand the challenges of living with cancer.

Community Organisations: Local or national organisations dedicated to cancer support, advocacy, and education offer resources such as educational materials, financial assistance programs, and wellness activities. Engaging with these organisations can provide additional avenues for support and empowerment.

Benefits of a Support Network:

Emotional Well-Being: Having supportive relationships can reduce stress, anxiety, and feelings of loneliness. Emotional well-being is crucial for maintaining resilience and coping effectively with the emotional rollercoaster of cancer treatment.

Practical Support: Supportive networks can assist with practical needs such as childcare, meal preparation, transportation, and navigating healthcare logistics. This practical assistance allows patients to focus more fully on their treatment and recovery.

Information and Advocacy: Members of a support network can help gather information about treatment options, clinical trials, and supportive care resources. They can also advocate on behalf of the patient to ensure their voice is heard in medical decision-making processes.

Be open about your needs and preferences with your support network. Communicate clearly how they can best help you—whether it's through companionship, practical assistance, or emotional support. While support is crucial, remember to establish boundaries and prioritise self-care. Clearly define the type and extent of support you require and communicate these limits respectfully with your network. If you find it challenging to establish or maintain a support network, consider seeking advice from a social worker, counsellor, or support group facilitator. These professionals can offer strategies and resources to strengthen your support system.

Building a support network is a cornerstone of effective cancer care. By surrounding oneself with supportive individuals and engaging with community resources, individuals affected by cancer can enhance their emotional well-being, access practical assistance, and cultivate a sense of empowerment throughout their cancer journey.

76. Reducing Environmental Toxins: Minimising Exposure to Pollutants

Exposure to environmental toxins and pollutants has been linked to various health risks, including cancer. While genetics, lifestyle factors, and medical history play significant roles in cancer development, reducing exposure to environmental toxins is an important aspect of cancer prevention and overall health maintenance. Adopting practices that minimise exposure to harmful substances can contribute to reducing the risk of cancer and supporting overall well-being.

Understanding Environmental Toxins:

Environmental toxins refer to substances found in the air, water, soil, and consumer products that have the potential to cause harm to human health. These toxins include pollutants from industrial emissions, pesticides, heavy metals, and chemicals found in everyday products such as cleaning agents, personal care products, and food packaging materials.

Exposure to environmental toxins has been linked to an increased risk of cancer, respiratory diseases, neurological disorders, reproductive issues, and other chronic health conditions. These substances can enter the body through inhalation, ingestion, and skin absorption, accumulating over time and potentially disrupting cellular functions and contributing to disease development.

Strategies to Minimise Exposure:

Air Quality: Improve indoor air quality by reducing exposure to indoor pollutants such as volatile organic compounds (VOCs) from paints, carpets, and cleaning products. Use air purifiers and ensure adequate ventilation in living and working spaces.

Water Quality: Drink filtered water to reduce exposure to contaminants such as chlorine, fluoride, and heavy metals that may be present in tap water. Consider installing water filtration systems at home to remove impurities.

Avoiding Pesticides: Choose organic produce whenever possible to minimise exposure to pesticides used in conventional farming practices. Wash fruits and vegetables thoroughly to remove residues before consumption.

Reducing Chemical Exposures: Use natural and eco-friendly household cleaning products, cosmetics, and personal care items that are free from harmful chemicals such as parabens, phthalates, and synthetic fragrances.

Safe Food Storage: Store food in glass containers or stainless steel instead of plastic containers to reduce exposure to potentially harmful chemicals like bisphenol A (BPA) and phthalates leaching into food.

Safe Handling of Hazardous Materials: Follow safety guidelines and wear protective gear when handling hazardous materials such as paints, solvents, and pesticides. Dispose of these substances properly according to local regulations.

Promoting stricter environmental regulations, endorsing sustainable practices, and engaging in community initiatives to curb pollution are pivotal in safeguarding public health and environmental integrity. By fostering awareness and championing cleaner environments, individuals contribute actively to minimising exposure to environmental toxins. While total elimination of such exposure may be challenging, making informed lifestyle choices and advocating for environmental responsibility can markedly decrease health risks for individuals and communities alike. Seeking advice from healthcare professionals and environmental specialists can offer personalised strategies to minimise exposure and foster healthier living conditions.

Minimising exposure to environmental toxins is a proactive step in cancer prevention and overall health promotion. By adopting practices that prioritise environmental stewardship and reducing personal exposure to harmful substances, individuals can contribute to a healthier future and support efforts in reducing cancer incidence and improving quality of life.

77. Relocating: Moving to a Healthier Environment

For individuals diagnosed with cancer, the environment in which they live can significantly impact their health and well-being. In some cases, considering relocation to a healthier environment may be a proactive decision to reduce exposure to environmental toxins, improve access to medical care, or enhance overall quality of life during cancer treatment and recovery.

Reasons for Considering Relocation:

Reducing Environmental Toxins: Moving to an area with cleaner air quality, lower levels of pollution, and reduced exposure to environmental toxins can potentially lower health risks associated with cancer and other chronic illnesses. This may be particularly beneficial for individuals sensitive to pollutants or those living in areas with high industrial or agricultural activity.

Access to Specialised Medical Care: Relocating to a region with renowned healthcare facilities, specialised cancer treatment centres, or clinical trial opportunities can provide access to advanced medical treatments, expert oncologists, and supportive care services tailored to individual needs.

Quality of Life Improvements: Moving to a community with a supportive network of family and friends, accessible recreational activities, and cultural amenities can enhance overall well-being and provide emotional support during the challenges of cancer treatment.

Stress Reduction: A change in environment, such as relocating to a quieter neighbourhood or closer to nature, can reduce stress levels and promote relaxation, which is beneficial for mental health and overall healing.

Discuss with healthcare providers, oncologists, and specialists to explore the potential advantages and drawbacks of moving based on individual health requirements, treatment schedules, and medical considerations. Assess financial implications, including healthcare expenses, insurance coverage, and cost of living adjustments in the prospective area. Take into account practical considerations such as job opportunities, housing availability, and proximity to support systems. Research local communities and available resources in the new location, such as cancer support groups, wellness initiatives, and community services that can aid in the transition and ongoing support. Familiarise yourself with legal obligations like residency criteria, healthcare accessibility, and necessary documentation, especially if relocating internationally.

Relocating is a deeply personal decision that should be based on individual circumstances, preferences, and medical advice. While it may offer potential health benefits, it's important to weigh the practical, emotional, and financial implications before making a decision. Some individuals may find that improving their current living environment through targeted interventions, such as air filtration systems or lifestyle changes, can also contribute to reducing environmental exposures and enhancing overall well-being.

Relocating to a healthier environment can be a strategic step towards optimising health outcomes and quality of life for individuals facing cancer. By carefully evaluating the potential benefits and challenges, consulting with healthcare professionals, and considering personal priorities, individuals can make informed decisions that support their cancer treatment journey and long-term well-being.

78. Decluttering: Reducing Stress by Organising Living Spaces

Decluttering involves the intentional process of simplifying and organising living environments to create a more harmonious and stress-free space. For individuals diagnosed with cancer, maintaining a clutter-free living environment can have significant psychological, emotional, and practical benefits that support overall well-being during treatment and recovery.

Psychological Benefits of Decluttering:

Stress Reduction: Cluttered spaces can contribute to feelings of overwhelm and stress. By decluttering, individuals can create a calming environment that promotes relaxation and mental clarity, which is essential for managing the emotional challenges associated with cancer diagnosis and treatment.

Enhanced Mood: A tidy and organised living space can positively impact mood and emotional well-being. Removing excess items and organising belongings can create a sense of order and control, fostering a more positive outlook and reducing feelings of anxiety or depression.

Improved Focus and Productivity: Clearing clutter can improve concentration and productivity levels. This is particularly beneficial for individuals managing treatment schedules, medication routines, and healthcare appointments, allowing them to focus on self-care and recovery.

Arranging living spaces ensures that necessary items are readily accessible, minimising the risk of accidents during periods of physical weakness or fatigue common during cancer treatment. Optimising living space by reducing clutter enhances functionality and comfort. This includes implementing efficient storage solutions, designating areas for relaxation or activities, and adjusting the environment to suit evolving health needs. A clutter-free home environment facilitates easier navigation for caregivers and support networks, improving their ability to provide assistance. Clear pathways and organised spaces simplify caregiving tasks and enhance overall efficiency in caregiving responsibilities.

Steps to Effective Decluttering:

Set Clear Goals: Define specific areas or rooms to declutter and establish achievable timelines and objectives. Prioritise spaces that are frequently used or contribute most to daily stress.

Sort and Simplify: Divide belongings into categories (keep, donate, discard) based on utility, sentimental value, or necessity. Consider the KonMari method or other organising principles to guide decision-making.

Organisational Systems: Implement storage solutions such as bins, shelves, and cabinets to maintain order and maximise space efficiency. Label containers and designate specific areas for different items to facilitate easy retrieval.

Maintenance and Sustainability: Establish habits for maintaining a clutter-free environment, such as regular cleaning routines, minimising new acquisitions, and periodically reassessing organisational systems.

Decluttering can evoke emotional responses, particularly when letting go of sentimental items or possessions with personal significance. It's important to approach decluttering with compassion and allow oneself time to process emotions associated with belongings.

Decluttering is more than just organising physical spaces—it's a transformative process that promotes emotional well-being, reduces stress, and enhances overall quality of life for individuals navigating the challenges of cancer treatment and recovery. By creating a supportive and organised living environment, individuals can cultivate a sense of peace, resilience, and empowerment as they focus on healing and maintaining optimal health.

Alternative Medical Systems

79. Anthroposophic Medicine: Integrating Spiritual and Physical Health

Anthroposophic Medicine is a holistic approach to healthcare that integrates spiritual, psychological, and physical aspects of healing. Developed by Rudolf Steiner in the early 20th century, this alternative medical system is based on the principles of anthroposophy, which emphasizes the interconnectedness of spiritual life and the natural world. Anthroposophic Medicine aims to treat the whole person—body, mind, and spirit—by enhancing the body's self-healing capacities and promoting overall well-being.

Principles of Anthroposophic Medicine:

Holistic Perspective: Anthroposophic Medicine views health as a dynamic balance between the physical body, life forces (or vital forces), and spiritual essence. It considers illness as an imbalance that affects the whole person and seeks to restore harmony through individualized treatment approaches.

Integration of Natural Therapies: Treatment modalities in Anthroposophic Medicine often include natural remedies derived from plants, minerals, and metals. These remedies are prepared according to specific anthroposophic pharmaceutical guidelines and are believed to support the body's innate healing processes.

Spiritual and Psychological Insights: Anthroposophic practitioners consider the spiritual and psychological dimensions of illness and health. They may use therapies such as counselling, art therapy, eurythmy (a movement therapy), and music therapy to address emotional and spiritual aspects that contribute to physical well-being.

Individualised Treatment Plans: Treatment in Anthroposophic Medicine is personalized to each individual's unique constitution, health history, and spiritual development. Practitioners assess the patient's physical symptoms alongside their emotional and spiritual state to tailor interventions accordingly.

Anthroposophic Medicine complements conventional cancer treatments by prioritizing the patient's well-being and resilience throughout treatment. Natural remedies and therapies are employed to alleviate symptoms like pain, fatigue, nausea, and anxiety associated with cancer. Mistletoe preparations, such as Iscador, are commonly used in Anthroposophic Cancer Therapy to support immune function and enhance overall health. This approach acknowledges the emotional and psychological impact of cancer, offering therapies like art therapy, eurythmy, and counseling as outlets for healing and emotional coping. Collaboration between Anthroposophic practitioners and oncologists ensures safe integration of complementary therapies, aiming to optimize treatment outcomes and improve the patient's overall care experience.

Critics of Anthroposophic Medicine raise concerns about its reliance on spiritual and esoteric principles that lack scientific validation. Skeptics argue that some therapies may lack empirical evidence of efficacy and safety, urging caution in their use as primary treatments for serious medical conditions like cancer.

Anthroposophic Medicine offers a holistic approach to cancer care that integrates spiritual, psychological, and physical dimensions of healing. While its principles align with patient-centered care and personalized treatment approaches, individuals considering Anthroposophic therapies should consult with qualified practitioners and discuss treatment options with their healthcare team.

80. Bioenergetics: Addressing Energy Imbalances

Bioenergetics is a branch of alternative medicine that focuses on the flow and balance of energy within the body. It operates on the principle that disruptions or imbalances in the body's energy pathways can contribute to illness, including cancer. Bioenergetic practitioners believe that restoring proper energy flow can support the body's natural healing mechanisms and promote overall health.

Principles of Bioenergetics:

Energy Systems: Bioenergetics is rooted in the concept of subtle energy systems that exist beyond the physical body. These systems include meridians (energy channels), chakras (energy centres), and the biofield (the electromagnetic field surrounding the body). Practitioners assess these energy systems to identify blockages or disruptions that may impact health.

Energy Healing Techniques: Bioenergetic therapies aim to rebalance and harmonize energy flow through various techniques, such as:

Acupuncture and Acupressure: Based on Traditional Chinese Medicine (TCM) principles, acupuncture involves inserting fine needles into specific points along meridians to stimulate energy flow and promote healing. Acupressure uses pressure on these points to achieve similar effects.

Reiki and Healing Touch: These practices involve the transfer of healing energy from the practitioner's hands to the patient's body to promote relaxation, reduce stress, and support overall well-being.

Biofield Therapies: Techniques like therapeutic touch and Qigong involve manipulating the biofield to remove energy blockages and restore balance.

Holistic Approach: Bioenergetics views health as a dynamic interaction between physical, emotional, mental, and spiritual aspects. Practitioners consider the interconnectedness of these dimensions and their influence on energy flow and overall vitality.

Bioenergetic approaches are integrated into cancer care to complement conventional treatments and promote holistic well-being. Techniques like acupuncture and acupressure are utilized to alleviate symptoms such as pain, nausea, fatigue, and insomnia, particularly during chemotherapy and radiation therapy. Additionally, biofield therapies such as Reiki and healing touch are employed to induce relaxation, reduce stress levels, and aid in managing the emotional and psychological impacts of cancer. These therapies aim to restore energy balance, strengthen the immune system, and bolster the body's innate defenses against cancer cells.

Bioenergetic therapies are frequently employed complementarily alongside conventional cancer treatments. Healthcare providers often suggest these therapies to alleviate treatment side effects, improve life quality, and enhance overall treatment effectiveness. Close collaboration between bioenergetic practitioners and oncology teams ensures patients receive coordinated and safe care. However, critics of bioenergetics contend that its concepts of energy flow and healing lack scientific validation. Skeptics question the efficacy and safety of bioenergetic therapies as primary treatments for serious medical conditions such as cancer. Healthcare providers stress the importance of evidence-based practices and advise patients to consult their oncologist before integrating bioenergetic therapies into their treatment regimen.

Bioenergetics offers a holistic approach to cancer care by addressing energy imbalances and promoting overall well-being through gentle, non-invasive techniques. While its principles may diverge from conventional medical practices, bioenergetic therapies have the potential to complement standard cancer treatments and support patients on their healing journey

Legal and Advocacy Actions

81. Seeking Second Opinions: Consulting Multiple Specialists

Seeking second opinions is a critical step in navigating a cancer diagnosis and treatment plan. It involves consulting with additional healthcare professionals to obtain different perspectives and recommendations regarding diagnosis, treatment options, and prognosis. This proactive approach empowers patients to make informed decisions about their care and ensures that they receive comprehensive evaluations from experts in the field.

Importance of Seeking Second Opinions:

Confirmation of Diagnosis: Cancer diagnoses can be complex, and different specialists may have varying interpretations of test results and clinical findings. Seeking a second opinion can provide reassurance and confirmation of the initial diagnosis, reducing uncertainty and potential misdiagnosis.

Exploration of Treatment Options: Cancer treatment plans may vary based on the expertise and experience of different oncologists and specialists. Consulting multiple specialists allows patients to explore various treatment approaches, including surgery, chemotherapy, radiation therapy, immunotherapy, targeted therapy, and clinical trials.

Risk Assessment and Prognosis: Second opinions can help patients understand the potential risks, benefits, and outcomes associated with different treatment options. Specialists may offer insights into prognosis, survival rates, and quality of life considerations, enabling patients to weigh their treatment decisions more comprehensively.

Personalised Care Plans: Each cancer case is unique, and treatment plans should be tailored to individual circumstances, preferences, and medical histories. Second opinions contribute to the development of personalised care plans that align with the patient's goals and priorities for treatment.

Patients seeking second opinions can start by researching reputable cancer centres and specialists recognised for their expertise in treating specific types of cancer. Referrals from primary care physicians, oncologists, or trusted healthcare providers can also guide the selection of specialists. To facilitate the second opinion consultation, patients should gather and organise their medical records, including pathology reports, imaging studies (such as CT scans and MRIs), and laboratory test results. Providing comprehensive information ensures specialists have a complete understanding of the patient's health status and prior treatments. During the consultation, patients are encouraged to inquire about the specialist's experience, treatment recommendations, potential side effects, and long-term outcomes. Open communication fosters a collaborative approach to decision-making, empowering patients to actively participate in their care journey.

Seeking second opinions is not only a patient's right but is also upheld by medical ethics and healthcare regulations. Healthcare systems and insurance providers typically cover the costs of second opinion consultations, recognising the significance of informed decision-making and thorough care planning. Patient advocacy organisations and support groups often provide resources and guidance to individuals navigating the second opinion process, aiming to facilitate access to top-quality healthcare and empower patients to advocate for their health needs and treatment preferences.

Seeking second opinions is a proactive and informed decision-making strategy for individuals facing a cancer diagnosis. By consulting multiple specialists, patients can gain clarity, explore treatment options, and develop personalised care plans that align with their medical needs and preferences. Embracing a collaborative approach to healthcare empowers patients to make well-informed decisions and enhances their overall experience of cancer care and treatment.

82. Patient Advocacy: Ensuring Patient Rights and Support

Patient advocacy plays a pivotal role in cancer care by safeguarding patient rights, promoting access to quality healthcare, and providing support throughout the cancer journey. Advocates work tirelessly to empower patients, enhance communication with healthcare providers, and advocate for policies that improve the overall patient experience and outcomes.

Navigating a cancer diagnosis and treatment journey can be daunting, involving intricate medical decisions and emotional hurdles. Patient advocates play a crucial role in guiding individuals through the healthcare system, offering essential information, resources, and support to help them navigate their care journey with confidence. They educate patients about their rights, treatment options, potential risks, and benefits, empowering them to actively participate in decision-making processes. Patient advocates ensure healthcare providers obtain informed consent before initiating treatments or procedures, collaborating closely with medical teams to address barriers to care such as insurance complexities, financial strains, and logistical challenges. They advocate for timely access to diagnostic tests, treatments, clinical trials, and supportive services tailored to the unique needs of cancer patients. Recognising the emotional toll of cancer, patient advocates also provide compassionate support, linking individuals with counseling services, support groups, and complementary therapies that foster well-being and resilience throughout treatment and recovery.

Advocacy Strategies and Initiatives:

Policy Advocacy: Patient advocates work with lawmakers, healthcare organisations, and regulatory agencies to shape policies that promote cancer research funding, access to innovative treatments, and equitable healthcare services. They champion legislative efforts to improve healthcare delivery, reduce disparities, and enhance patient outcomes.

Community Engagement: Advocacy organisations and support networks offer platforms for patients, caregivers, and healthcare professionals to share experiences, raise awareness about cancer-related issues, and advocate for improved care standards within local communities and nationwide.

Educational Outreach: Patient advocates develop educational resources, workshops, and conferences that empower individuals with cancer-related knowledge, skills, and strategies to navigate their healthcare journeys confidently. They foster informed decision-making and promote health literacy among diverse populations affected by cancer.

Effective patient advocacy hinges on collaborative partnerships with healthcare providers, including oncologists, nurses, social workers, and other allied professionals. By nurturing transparent communication and mutual respect, advocates ensure that patient preferences, priorities, and apprehensions are woven into cohesive care strategies. Upholding stringent confidentiality norms, advocates safeguard patients' medical data and uphold their right to privacy throughout the advocacy journey. Advocates prioritise informed consent, ensuring patients comprehend the ramifications of treatment choices and have ample opportunity to inquire and gather supplementary details before consenting to medical interventions.

Patient advocacy is a cornerstone of cancer care, advocating for patient rights, promoting informed decision-making, and enhancing the overall quality of life for individuals affected by cancer. By providing support, resources, and advocacy initiatives, patient advocates empower patients to navigate their healthcare journeys with confidence, resilience, and dignity.

83. Legal Medical Cannabis: Using Legal Cannabis for Symptom Management

Legal medical cannabis, also known as medical marijuana, refers to the use of cannabis or cannabinoids under medical supervision to alleviate symptoms associated with cancer and its treatments. As attitudes and regulations surrounding cannabis evolve, many cancer patients explore cannabis as a complementary therapy to manage pain, nausea, appetite loss, insomnia, and other side effects of cancer therapies.

Benefits of Legal Medical Cannabis:

Pain Management: Cannabis contains compounds such as THC (tetrahydrocannabinol) and CBD (cannabidiol) that interact with the body's endocannabinoid system, potentially reducing pain intensity and improving pain relief for cancer patients, especially those experiencing neuropathic pain.

Nausea and Vomiting: Cannabis has antiemetic properties that can help alleviate chemotherapy-induced nausea and vomiting, which are common side effects that can significantly impact a patient's quality of life.

Appetite Stimulation: Cancer treatments often lead to appetite loss and weight loss. Cannabis may stimulate appetite and promote weight gain in patients undergoing chemotherapy or radiation therapy, potentially improving nutritional intake and overall well-being.

Sleep Disturbances: Insomnia and sleep disturbances are prevalent among cancer patients. Certain strains of cannabis may have sedative effects, aiding in sleep induction and improving sleep quality.

Anxiety and Mood Disorders: Cancer diagnosis and treatment can lead to anxiety, depression, and mood disorders. CBD, a non-psychoactive compound in cannabis, has shown promise in reducing anxiety symptoms and promoting relaxation.

Legal Considerations and Regulatory Framework:

Medical Cannabis Programs: Many countries and states have established medical cannabis programs that regulate the cultivation, distribution, and use of cannabis for medical purposes. Patients may need to obtain a medical cannabis card or prescription from a qualified healthcare provider to legally access cannabis products.

Dosage and Administration: Medical cannabis is available in various forms, including dried flowers for smoking or vaporisation, oils, tinctures, edibles, and topical creams. Healthcare providers can recommend appropriate dosages and administration methods based on the patient's symptoms, medical history, and treatment goals.

Safety and Side Effects: While cannabis may offer therapeutic benefits, it is essential to consider potential side effects, drug interactions, and safety concerns. Patients should disclose their cannabis use to healthcare providers to ensure coordinated care and monitor for adverse effects.

Patient advocacy organisations serve a pivotal role in advancing access to medical cannabis, advocating for broader legalisation, and combating the stigma surrounding cannabis within medical contexts. These groups offer educational materials and support to aid patients and caregivers in navigating legal landscapes, comprehending the potential advantages and drawbacks of medical cannabis, and making well-informed choices regarding its integration into cancer treatment regimens.

Legal medical cannabis represents a complementary approach to managing symptoms associated with cancer and its treatments. By harnessing the therapeutic potential of cannabis under medical supervision, cancer patients may experience relief from pain, nausea, appetite loss, and other treatment-related side effects, ultimately enhancing their quality of life and well-being.

Innovative and Cutting-Edge Therapies

84. Oncolytic Viruses: Using Viruses to Target Cancer Cells

Oncolytic viruses represent a groundbreaking approach in cancer treatment, harnessing the natural ability of viruses to selectively infect and destroy cancer cells while sparing healthy tissues. These viruses are engineered or naturally occurring viruses that are modified to specifically target and kill cancer cells, offering a promising avenue for overcoming the challenges of conventional treatments.

Oncolytic viruses are engineered to exploit the unique biology of cancer cells. They are designed to identify specific receptors or molecular markers on the surface of these cells, enabling them to selectively infect and replicate within tumours. Once inside, the viruses replicate, causing the cancer cells to lyse (break open) and release viral particles that can then infect nearby cancer cells. This amplifies the therapeutic effect, potentially leading to extensive cancer cell death. Beyond directly killing cancer cells, oncolytic viruses also stimulate the immune system to respond against the tumour. The viral infection releases danger signals and tumour antigens, activating immune cells like T cells and natural killer (NK) cells to recognise and attack cancer cells throughout the body.

Types of Oncolytic Viruses:

Adenoviruses: Adenoviruses are common viruses that cause respiratory infections in humans. They have been modified to carry therapeutic genes or to replicate selectively in cancer cells.

Herpes Simplex Viruses (HSV): HSV, the virus responsible for cold sores, has been engineered to replicate in and destroy cancer cells. It has shown promise in clinical trials for treating various cancers, including melanoma and glioblastoma.

Reoviruses: Reoviruses are naturally occurring viruses that preferentially replicate in cancer cells with activated Ras signalling pathways, which are common in many types of cancer.

Vaccinia Virus: The vaccinia virus, used in smallpox vaccination, has been adapted to selectively replicate in and destroy cancer cells while leaving healthy cells unharmed.

Oncolytic viruses have been tested in clinical trials for various cancers, including melanoma, glioblastoma, breast cancer, and pancreatic cancer. These trials assess the safety, efficacy, and optimal dosing of oncolytic viruses both as monotherapies and in combination with other treatments. Researchers are investigating combinations of oncolytic viruses with chemotherapy, radiation therapy, and immunotherapy to enhance treatment responses and overcome resistance mechanisms in cancer cells. Advances in genetic sequencing and molecular profiling enable personalised approaches to oncolytic virus therapy, focusing on tumour-specific modifications and patient-specific immune responses to improve treatment outcomes and minimise side effects.

Challenges and Future Directions:

Immune Response and Resistance: Some patients may develop immune responses against the oncolytic virus, limiting its effectiveness. Researchers are investigating strategies to enhance viral persistence and immune evasion within the tumour microenvironment.

Safety and Toxicity: Ensuring the safety of oncolytic viruses is critical, as viral replication within the body can potentially lead to systemic side effects. Ongoing research focuses on optimising viral delivery methods and minimising off-target effects.

Regulatory Approval: Despite promising preclinical and clinical results, the approval process for oncolytic viruses involves rigorous evaluation of safety, efficacy, and manufacturing standards by regulatory agencies worldwide.

Oncolytic viruses represent a transformative approach in cancer therapy, leveraging the inherent properties of viruses to target and destroy cancer cells while stimulating an immune response against the tumour. As research advances and clinical trials continue to demonstrate promising results, oncolytic viruses hold the potential to become a valuable addition to the armamentarium of cancer treatments, offering hope for improved outcomes and quality of life for patients fighting cancer.

85. Photodynamic Therapy: Using Light-Activated Drugs

Photodynamic therapy (PDT) is a non-invasive treatment modality that harnesses the power of light and photosensitive drugs (photosensitizers) to selectively destroy cancer cells while minimising damage to surrounding healthy tissue. This therapy offers a targeted approach to treating various types of cancer and has shown promising results in clinical settings.

The first step in photodynamic therapy (PDT) involves administering a photosensitising agent either orally or intravenously, which selectively accumulates in cancer cells over time. Once the photosensitizer has sufficiently built up in the tumour tissue, specific wavelengths of light are externally applied to the tumour area. This light activates the photosensitizer, prompting it to produce reactive oxygen species (ROS) and other cytotoxic molecules. These reactive oxygen species induce oxidative stress within the cancer cells, damaging proteins, lipids, and DNA. This process ultimately results in apoptosis, or programmed cell death, of the cancer cells.

PDT has been employed to treat various cancers, including skin cancers (basal cell carcinoma and squamous cell carcinoma), lung cancer, oesophageal cancer, bladder cancer, and certain head and neck cancers. PDT offers several advantages over traditional cancer therapies: it is minimally invasive, allows for precise targeting of cancerous tissue, preserves surrounding healthy tissue, and presents a lower risk of systemic side effects compared to chemotherapy and radiation therapy. Researchers are investigating the use of PDT in combination with other treatments such as surgery, chemotherapy, and immunotherapy to enhance its effectiveness and improve patient outcomes.

Technological Advances:

Light Delivery Systems: Advances in light delivery systems have improved the precision and depth of light penetration into tumour tissues, allowing for more effective treatment of deeper-seated tumours.

Photosensitizer Development: Ongoing research focuses on developing new photosensitizers with enhanced targeting capabilities, improved tumour selectivity, and optimised pharmacokinetic properties to enhance PDT efficacy.

Imaging and Monitoring: Real-time imaging techniques, such as fluorescence imaging and spectroscopy, are being integrated into PDT procedures to visualise the distribution of photosensitizers within tumours and monitor treatment response.

Challenges and Considerations:

Light Penetration: The effectiveness of PDT is limited by the depth to which light can penetrate tissue. Researchers are exploring strategies to overcome this limitation, such as using fibre optic devices and light-emitting diodes (LEDs) for light delivery.

Photosensitivity: Patients undergoing PDT may experience temporary sensitivity to light, requiring precautions to minimise sun exposure and artificial light sources for a period following treatment.

Clinical Implementation: PDT's integration into clinical practice requires standardised protocols, training of healthcare providers, and continued evaluation through clinical trials to optimise treatment outcomes and ensure patient safety.

Photodynamic therapy represents a promising approach in cancer treatment, leveraging light-activated drugs to selectively target and destroy cancer cells while preserving surrounding healthy tissue. As research and technological advancements continue to refine PDT protocols and expand its applications across different cancer types, PDT holds significant potential to improve treatment outcomes and quality of life for patients battling cancer.

86. Thermal Ablation: Destroying Tumours with Heat

Thermal ablation is a minimally invasive technique used to destroy tumours by applying localised heat directly to cancerous tissue. This innovative therapy offers an alternative to surgery for treating small tumours in various organs and has demonstrated efficacy in clinical settings.

Thermal ablation techniques, which include radiofrequency ablation (RFA), microwave ablation (MWA), laser ablation (LA), and high-intensity focused ultrasound (HIFU), use various energy sources to generate heat and induce coagulative necrosis (cell death) within tumours. During thermal ablation, a probe or applicator is inserted into the tumour under imaging guidance (such as ultrasound or CT scan) to precisely target the cancerous tissue. Once positioned, the energy source (radiofrequency waves, microwaves, laser light, or focused ultrasound waves) is applied to heat and destroy the tumour cells. Thermal ablation is particularly effective for treating small tumours (typically less than 3-5 cm in diameter) in organs such as the liver, kidney, lung, and bone. Additionally, it can be used to relieve symptoms and improve the quality of life for patients with advanced cancer who are not candidates for surgery.

Clinical Applications:

Liver Cancer: Thermal ablation is widely used for treating primary liver tumours (hepatocellular carcinoma) and metastatic liver lesions from colorectal cancer and other primary cancers.

Lung Cancer: In select cases, thermal ablation can be used to treat early-stage lung cancers or metastatic lung nodules, providing a less invasive alternative to surgical resection.

Renal Cancer: For small kidney tumours (renal cell carcinoma), thermal ablation has shown comparable efficacy to surgical removal (nephrectomy) while preserving kidney function.

Bone Metastases: Thermal ablation techniques, particularly radiofrequency and microwave ablation, are utilised to palliate painful bone metastases and improve mobility.

Thermal ablation procedures are performed using small incisions or percutaneous approaches, minimising trauma to surrounding healthy tissue and reducing recovery time compared to surgery. By targeting and destroying tumours while sparing healthy tissue, thermal ablation helps preserve organ function and can be repeated if new tumours develop. Additionally, thermal ablation can be combined with other treatment modalities such as chemotherapy, immunotherapy, and targeted therapy to enhance treatment outcomes and address residual disease.

Advances in imaging technologies, such as MRI-guided and CT-guided systems, have significantly improved the accuracy of tumour targeting and the precise delivery of thermal energy to the tumour site. Real-time monitoring techniques, including temperature sensors and thermal imaging, allow healthcare providers to track tissue temperatures during ablation procedures and adjust energy delivery as needed to optimise treatment outcomes. Ongoing clinical trials are exploring the application of thermal ablation for new cancer types, refining techniques, and comparing its efficacy with standard treatments to expand its therapeutic potential.

Challenges and Considerations:

Tumour Size and Location: The effectiveness of thermal ablation may be limited by tumour size, location near critical structures, and heat dissipation in larger tumours.

Post-Treatment Monitoring: Patients undergoing thermal ablation require regular follow-up imaging to assess treatment response, detect recurrence, and manage potential complications such as post-procedural pain or fluid accumulation.

Patient Selection: Careful patient selection based on tumour characteristics, location, and overall health is crucial to achieving optimal outcomes with thermal ablation.

Thermal ablation represents an innovative and minimally invasive approach to treating cancer, utilising heat-based technologies to destroy tumours while preserving organ function and improving patient quality of life. As research and technological advancements continue to enhance the precision, safety, and efficacy of thermal ablation techniques, this therapy holds promise as a valuable tool in the multidisciplinary treatment of cancer.

87. Magnetic Hyperthermia: Using Magnetic Fields to Heat and Kill Cancer Cells

Magnetic hyperthermia is an emerging therapy that utilises magnetic nanoparticles (MNPs) to selectively heat and destroy cancer cells within tumours. This non-invasive approach shows promise in targeting tumours while minimising damage to surrounding healthy tissues.

Magnetic nanoparticles, often made from materials like iron oxide, are either injected into the bloodstream or directly into the tumour site. These nanoparticles selectively accumulate in the tumour due to the enhanced permeability and retention (EPR) effect. Once localised within the tumour tissue, an alternating magnetic field (AMF) is applied externally. This AMF causes the magnetic nanoparticles to oscillate rapidly, generating heat through hysteresis and relaxation mechanisms. The heat produced induces hyperthermia (elevated temperature) specifically within the tumour cells. Cancer cells are more susceptible to heat-induced damage than normal cells because of their altered metabolism and impaired heat dissipation. Elevated temperatures (typically between 40-45°C) disrupt cellular membranes, denature proteins, and activate apoptotic pathways in cancer cells, leading to cell death. Additionally, localised hyperthermia can enhance the effectiveness of concurrent treatments like chemotherapy and radiation therapy.

Clinical Applications:

Brain Tumours: Magnetic hyperthermia is being investigated for the treatment of glioblastoma and other brain tumours, where traditional therapies face challenges due to the blood-brain barrier.

Breast Cancer: Studies have explored magnetic hyperthermia as a potential treatment for breast cancer, including both primary tumours and metastatic lesions.

Prostate Cancer: Research has shown promise in using magnetic hyperthermia to target prostate cancer cells, particularly in combination with other localised treatments.

Magnetic hyperthermia allows for precise targeting of tumours using magnetic nanoparticles, which reduces damage to healthy tissues and minimises side effects compared to traditional therapies. This non-invasive procedure doesn't require surgery, making it suitable for patients who are not surgical candidates or have tumours in hard-to-reach areas. Additionally, hyperthermia can enhance the effectiveness of chemotherapy and radiation therapy by increasing drug uptake and radiosensitivity in cancer cells.

Technological Advances:

Nanoparticle Design: Advances in nanoparticle engineering aim to improve the biocompatibility, stability, and tumour-targeting specificity of magnetic nanoparticles.

Magnetic Field Optimisation: Ongoing research focuses on optimising the frequency, amplitude, and duration of the AMF to maximise heat generation within tumours while minimising off-target effects.

Imaging Integration: Magnetic resonance imaging (MRI) and other imaging modalities are integrated into magnetic hyperthermia procedures to monitor nanoparticle distribution, assess treatment response, and guide therapy adjustments.

Achieving effective delivery and accumulation of magnetic nanoparticles within tumours remains a significant challenge, especially for tumours that are deep-seated or heterogeneous in nature. Ongoing research is focused on investigating the safety of magnetic nanoparticles, including potential long-term effects and addressing biocompatibility concerns to ensure patient safety. Magnetic hyperthermia techniques are currently in investigational stages in many countries, necessitating rigorous clinical trials and regulatory approvals before they can be widely adopted for clinical use.

Magnetic hyperthermia represents a promising advancement in cancer treatment, leveraging magnetic nanoparticles and alternating magnetic fields to induce selective tumour heating and cell death. As research continues to refine nanoparticle design, optimise treatment protocols, and expand clinical applications, magnetic hyperthermia holds potential to enhance therapeutic outcomes and provide new options for patients facing challenging cancer diagnoses.

88. Optogenetics: Controlling Cells with Light (Experimental)

Optogenetics represents a pioneering technique that allows scientists to control cellular activity using light-sensitive proteins called opsins. While primarily used in neuroscience to manipulate neuronal activity, optogenetics is now being explored for its potential applications in cancer therapy, albeit still in experimental stages.

In integrating optogenetics into cancer therapy, scientists modify cancer cells or immune cells with opsins, light-sensitive proteins sourced from microorganisms such as algae and bacteria. Once opsins are embedded in the cellular membrane of target cells, they can be activated using particular wavelengths of light, often within the visible spectrum (e.g., blue or yellow light). Activation by light induces alterations in cellular behaviour and signalling pathways. By regulating light exposure, researchers can finely tune cellular activities such as proliferation, apoptosis (programmed cell death), migration, and modulation of immune responses.

Potential Applications in Cancer Treatment: In the context of cancer therapy, optogenetics holds several promising applications:

Gene Expression Control: Opsins can be used to control the expression of genes involved in cancer progression or immune response. This capability could potentially inhibit oncogenic pathways or enhance anti-tumour immune responses.

Selective Cell Killing: Light activation of opsins integrated into cancer cells can induce apoptosis or disrupt essential cellular functions, leading to selective tumour cell death.

Immunomodulation: Opsins expressed in immune cells could be activated to enhance their cytotoxic activity against cancer cells or regulate immune checkpoint pathways involved in tumour evasion.

Early investigations have demonstrated the potential of optogenetics in influencing cellular behaviour in laboratory settings and animal models of cancer. Researchers are actively exploring methods to improve the precision and effectiveness of optogenetic treatments through enhancements in opsin expression, advancements in light delivery systems, and integration with complementary therapies such as chemotherapy or immunotherapy. However, several challenges must be addressed before optogenetics can progress to clinical applications: Ensuring efficient delivery of opsins and light to tumour sites while minimising damage to surrounding tissues is paramount. The safety profile of opsins, potential immune responses they may provoke, and the long-term consequences of prolonged light exposure require rigorous evaluation. Regulatory pathways for experimental therapies like optogenetics necessitate thorough preclinical testing and clinical trials to establish their safety and efficacy.

Further progress in genetic engineering and synthetic biology will refine the accuracy and flexibility of optogenetic technologies in cancer therapy. Collaboration among researchers, clinicians, and regulatory bodies is crucial for navigating the path toward clinical application and their eventual incorporation into established cancer treatment protocols.

Optogenetics represents a groundbreaking approach in cancer research, leveraging light-sensitive proteins to control cellular behaviour and potentially revolutionise cancer therapy. While still in the experimental stage, ongoing research holds promise for expanding the therapeutic arsenal against cancer, offering new avenues for targeted, precise, and customisable treatments tailored to individual patients.

Personal and Spiritual Development

89. Mindfulness Meditation: Practicing Mindfulness to Reduce Stress

Mindfulness meditation has gained significant attention in recent years as a powerful practice for enhancing mental, emotional, and spiritual well-being. Rooted in ancient contemplative traditions, mindfulness involves intentionally focusing one's attention on the present moment without judgment. This practice has shown substantial benefits in reducing stress, managing pain, and improving overall quality of life, particularly for individuals navigating the challenges of cancer diagnosis and treatment.

Benefits of Mindfulness Meditation:

Stress Reduction: Cancer diagnosis and treatment can lead to significant stress and anxiety. Mindfulness meditation offers a structured approach to cultivate awareness of thoughts, emotions, and bodily sensations, thereby reducing psychological distress and promoting a sense of calm.

Pain Management: Chronic pain is a common issue for cancer patients. Mindfulness practices have been shown to enhance pain tolerance and decrease the perceived intensity of pain through non-reactive awareness and acceptance.

Emotional Regulation: Cancer often brings forth a range of intense emotions such as fear, anger, and sadness.

Mindfulness meditation helps individuals develop emotional resilience by fostering a compassionate and non-judgmental attitude towards their internal experiences.

Improved Sleep Quality: Many cancer patients struggle with sleep disturbances. Regular mindfulness practice has been linked to improved sleep patterns by promoting relaxation and reducing insomnia symptoms.

Enhanced Cognitive Function: Cancer treatments like chemotherapy can impact cognitive function, often referred to as "chemo brain." Mindfulness meditation may help mitigate cognitive decline by enhancing attention, memory, and cognitive flexibility.

Created by Dr. Jon Kabat-Zinn, Mindfulness-Based Stress Reduction (MBSR) is a structured program blending mindfulness meditation, yoga, and psychoeducation. It's extensively used in clinical settings to help cancer patients and survivors manage stressors associated with treatment. Mindfulness-Based Cognitive Therapy (MBCT) combines mindfulness practices with cognitive-behavioural techniques to prevent depression relapse and address mood disturbances during prolonged cancer treatment. Mindfulness promotes self-compassion by guiding individuals to approach their illness with kindness and acceptance, diminishing self-criticism and improving emotional health.

Regularly participating in mindfulness meditation sessions, usually lasting between 10 to 30 minutes, helps individuals develop present-moment awareness and enhance relaxation responses. Integrating mindfulness into daily routines, such as mindful eating, walking, or breathing exercises, supports ongoing awareness and stress reduction throughout the day.

Mindfulness meditation offers a space for individuals to connect with their inner wisdom, promoting spiritual growth and a deeper sense of meaning and purpose amid illness. Through mindfulness practice, cancer patients can cultivate resilience, empowering them to navigate uncertainties, treatment complexities, and life transitions with greater equanimity and grace.

Mindfulness meditation offers cancer patients and survivors a transformative practice for cultivating inner resilience, reducing stress, managing pain, and fostering spiritual and emotional well-being. Integrating mindfulness into cancer care not only supports psychological adjustment but also enhances overall quality of life, empowering individuals to face the journey of cancer treatment with greater peace and acceptance.

90. Journaling: Writing to Process Emotions

Journaling is a therapeutic practice that involves writing regularly to explore thoughts, emotions, and experiences. It serves as a powerful tool for individuals facing the challenges of cancer diagnosis, treatment, and survivorship, providing a structured way to process emotions, gain clarity, and promote personal growth and spiritual well-being.

Benefits of Journaling:

Emotional Expression: Cancer diagnosis often brings forth a whirlwind of emotions such as fear, anxiety, sadness, and anger. Journaling provides a safe space to express and release these emotions, reducing psychological distress and promoting emotional healing.

Clarity and Insight: Writing about experiences and reflections can offer insights into one's thoughts, behaviours, and coping mechanisms. It helps individuals gain perspective on their journey with cancer, uncovering underlying beliefs and patterns that may influence their emotional responses.

Stress Reduction: Chronic stress is a common companion throughout the cancer journey. Regular journaling has been shown to lower stress levels by providing an outlet for processing stressful events, organising thoughts, and problem-solving.

Enhanced Self-Awareness: Through journaling, individuals can deepen their understanding of themselves, their values, and their strengths. This self-awareness fosters personal growth and empowers individuals to make informed decisions about their health and well-being.

Promotion of Resilience: Writing about challenges and setbacks in a journal can help individuals reframe negative experiences, find meaning in adversity, and build resilience. It encourages a proactive approach to coping with the uncertainties of cancer treatment and recovery.

Allocating dedicated daily time for journaling enables individuals to process emotions in real-time, track their progress, and celebrate milestones throughout their cancer journey. Using prompts like "Today, I feel...", "I am grateful for...", or "My biggest fear about cancer is..." encourages deeper reflection and emotional exploration. Journaling can also serve as a tool for setting goals related to health, lifestyle adjustments, or personal growth. Consistently reviewing progress toward these goals fosters motivation and a sense of accomplishment.

Journaling supports introspection and deepens connection with personal spiritual beliefs, values, and sources of strength. It prompts individuals to ponder existential questions and discover meaning within their cancer journey. By integrating gratitude journaling or mindfulness practices into daily entries, individuals nurture an appreciation for life's positive aspects, fostering inner peace and acceptance amid adversity.

Exploring various journaling methods like free-writing, bullet journaling, or artistic expression through art or poetry can cater to personal preferences and amplify therapeutic benefits. Sharing journal entries with trusted loved ones, support groups, or therapists can also be valuable, fostering connections and mutual understanding.

Journaling is a profound tool for personal and spiritual development throughout the cancer journey, offering a structured means to process emotions, gain clarity, and cultivate resilience. By engaging in regular journaling practices, individuals can navigate the complexities of cancer diagnosis and treatment with greater emotional awareness, insight, and inner strength.

91. Yoga: Combining Physical and Mental Practices

Yoga is a holistic discipline that integrates physical postures (asanas), breath control (pranayama), meditation, and relaxation techniques. It originated in ancient India and has evolved into various styles and practices worldwide. In the context of cancer care, yoga serves as a powerful tool for enhancing physical well-being, managing treatment side effects, and promoting emotional and spiritual resilience.

Physical Benefits of Yoga:

Improved Flexibility and Strength: Cancer treatments such as chemotherapy and radiation can cause muscle stiffness and weakness. Yoga asanas gently stretch and strengthen muscles, joints, and connective tissues, improving flexibility and mobility.

Pain Management: Many cancer patients experience chronic pain due to tumours, surgery, or treatment side effects. Certain yoga postures and gentle movements can alleviate muscular tension, reduce pain perception, and enhance overall comfort.

Enhanced Energy Levels: Fatigue is a common side effect of cancer treatment. Practicing yoga helps increase circulation, oxygenation, and vitality, providing a natural energy boost without the harsh stimulants of caffeine or medications.

Support for Immune Function: Yoga practices such as twisting poses and gentle inversions stimulate lymphatic circulation, which supports immune system function and helps the body detoxify more effectively.

Coping with a cancer diagnosis and treatment often brings increased stress and anxiety. Yoga, with its meditative aspects and controlled breathing techniques (pranayama), promotes relaxation, reduces cortisol levels, and enhances emotional resilience. Many cancer patients experience insomnia and sleep disturbances, but yoga encourages relaxation, calms the mind, and supports better sleep patterns, promoting restorative rest. By cultivating mindfulness and present-moment awareness, yoga helps individuals manage emotional fluctuations, fear, and uncertainty related to cancer, fostering inner peace and emotional stability.

Yoga facilitates self-reflection and introspection, offering a sacred sanctuary for individuals to connect with their inner wisdom, values, and spiritual beliefs. It encourages exploration of existential questions and the quest for meaning in the midst of illness. Embracing the holistic approach of yoga promotes harmony among the physical body, mind, and spirit. With consistent practice, individuals often find a heightened sense of self-awareness, purpose, and a deeper connection to a higher power or universal consciousness.

Yoga can be tailored to meet the needs of individuals with varying physical abilities and at different stages of treatment. Gentle yoga, chair yoga, or restorative yoga sessions are particularly suitable for those recovering from surgery or undergoing intensive treatments. Participating in yoga classes or support groups designed specifically for cancer patients fosters a sense of community, mutual support, and empathy. It creates opportunities for social interaction and emotional healing.

Yoga is a holistic practice that addresses the physical, mental, emotional, and spiritual aspects of individuals affected by cancer. By incorporating yoga into their daily routine, cancer patients and survivors can experience improved physical functioning, reduced stress levels, enhanced emotional well-being, and deeper spiritual growth. Yoga empowers individuals to cultivate resilience, embrace healing, and foster a sense of wholeness amidst the challenges of cancer diagnosis and treatment.

92. Prayer: Engaging in Religious Practices

Prayer is a deeply personal and spiritual practice that holds profound significance for individuals facing cancer. Rooted in various religious and spiritual traditions worldwide, prayer involves the communication with a higher power or spiritual force through spoken words, thoughts, or contemplative silence. In the realm of cancer treatment and recovery, prayer serves as a powerful tool for cultivating inner strength, finding solace, and fostering hope amidst the challenges of the disease.

Spiritual Connection and Comfort

For many individuals diagnosed with cancer, prayer provides a source of comfort, reassurance, and a sense of spiritual connection during difficult times. It offers a means to express fears, hopes, and gratitude, and to seek guidance and peace. Engaging in communal prayer within religious communities or support groups can foster a sense of belonging and solidarity. It provides opportunities for mutual support, shared experiences, and collective healing prayers.

Emotional and Psychological Benefits

Stress Reduction: Cancer diagnosis and treatment can evoke intense emotional stress, anxiety, and uncertainty. Prayer promotes relaxation, reduces stress hormones like cortisol, and enhances emotional resilience. It encourages individuals to surrender worries and concerns to a higher power, thereby alleviating psychological burdens.

Coping with Fear and Uncertainty: Prayer helps individuals cope with fear of the unknown, mortality, and existential questions that arise with a cancer diagnosis. It offers a framework for processing emotions, finding meaning in suffering, and embracing acceptance.

Healing and Restoration:

Promoting Positive Outlook: Prayer cultivates a positive mindset and hopeful outlook, which are essential for navigating the challenges of cancer treatment and recovery. It encourages individuals to focus on healing, restoration, and the possibility of recovery.

Enhancing Spiritual Growth: Beyond physical healing, prayer fosters spiritual growth and transformation. It deepens individuals' connection to their faith, values, and beliefs, leading to a sense of spiritual fulfilment and purpose amidst adversity.

Prayer is versatile and can be customised according to personal beliefs, traditions, and preferences. Whether through structured religious rituals, spontaneous prayers, meditation, or reflective contemplation, individuals can personalise their prayer practices to resonate with their spiritual path and journey towards healing. Engaging in religious services, joining prayer groups, or attending spiritual retreats connects individuals with a supportive community of like-minded peers. These settings foster shared prayer intentions, intercessory prayers, and collective spiritual support.

Prayer is a profound and integral aspect of personal and spiritual development for individuals confronting cancer. It serves as a source of strength, solace, and spiritual guidance throughout the cancer journey. By engaging in prayer, individuals can cultivate inner peace, resilience, and a deeper connection to their faith, values, and sense of purpose. Prayer empowers individuals to navigate the physical, emotional, and spiritual dimensions of cancer with hope, courage, and a renewed sense of spiritual well-being.

93. Gratitude Practices: Focusing on Positive Aspects of Life

Gratitude practices involve intentionally focusing on and appreciating the positive aspects of life, even amidst challenges such as cancer. Cultivating gratitude is not merely about acknowledging blessings, but also about fostering a mindset that enhances emotional well-being, resilience, and spiritual growth. Incorporating gratitude into daily life can significantly impact how individuals navigate the complexities of cancer treatment and recovery.

Benefits of Gratitude Practices:

Emotional Resilience: Cancer diagnosis and treatment can evoke a wide range of emotions, including fear, sadness, and anxiety. Gratitude practices help individuals cultivate emotional resilience by shifting focus from difficulties to blessings. This shift in perspective promotes a positive outlook and enhances coping mechanisms.

Stress Reduction: Practicing gratitude has been linked to reduced levels of stress hormones like cortisol. By acknowledging and appreciating positive experiences, relationships, and moments of joy, individuals can mitigate the effects of stress associated with cancer.

Enhanced Well-being: Regular gratitude practices contribute to overall psychological well-being. They promote feelings of contentment, satisfaction, and happiness, even during challenging times. This emotional well-being is crucial for maintaining quality of life and supporting healing processes.

Gratitude practices prompt individuals to contemplate their values, priorities, and sources of life's meaning. By expressing gratitude for relationships, personal strengths, and moments of grace, people can strengthen their connection to their spiritual beliefs and sense of purpose. Cancer often raises profound existential questions and uncertainties. Gratitude practices aid in accepting life's complexities and assist individuals in finding peace amidst adversity. These practices cultivate a sense of trust in the unfolding journey, regardless of the outcomes.

Integrating gratitude into daily routines can be achieved through practices like maintaining a gratitude journal, expressing appreciation to loved ones, or contemplating blessings during meditation. These rituals serve as regular reminders of the abundance and positivity present in one's life. Sharing expressions of gratitude with caregivers, healthcare providers, and support networks strengthens relationships and cultivates mutual appreciation. This fosters a deepened sense of connection and underscores the vital role of community in the healing journey.

Gratitude practices are transformative tools for personal and spiritual development amidst the challenges of cancer. By focusing on positive aspects of life, acknowledging blessings, and nurturing a mindset of appreciation, individuals can enhance emotional resilience, promote well-being, and deepen their spiritual connection. Gratitude empowers individuals to navigate the complexities of cancer treatment with grace, optimism, and a profound sense of inner peace.

Community and Social Engagement

94. Public Speaking: Sharing Experiences to Inspire Others

Public speaking, particularly sharing personal experiences with cancer, can be a powerful form of community and social engagement. It involves individuals speaking openly and authentically about their cancer journey, challenges faced, lessons learned, and hopes for the future. By sharing their stories, individuals not only inspire and educate others but also contribute to raising awareness, fostering empathy, and building supportive communities.

Public speaking offers individuals a platform to inspire and uplift others navigating similar challenges. Through sharing stories of resilience, perseverance, and personal growth, speakers provide concrete examples of overcoming adversity and thriving despite cancer. These engagements also serve as opportunities to educate audiences on diverse aspects of cancer, ranging from symptoms and treatment options to the psychosocial impacts. By imparting this knowledge, speakers empower listeners to make informed health decisions and adopt proactive healthcare practices.

Public speaking events unite individuals impacted by cancer, caregivers, healthcare professionals, and members of the community. These gatherings cultivate connections, mutual understanding, and a shared sense of belonging within the cancer community. By openly sharing experiences with cancer, these events challenge misconceptions and diminish stigma associated with the disease. They foster a culture of empathy, compassion, and solidarity for individuals and families navigating the challenges of cancer.

Sharing one's cancer journey through public speaking fosters reflection and introspection. It provides individuals with a platform to process emotions, gain perspective on their experiences, and discover meaning in their journey. Public speaking empowers individuals to become advocates for themselves and others within the cancer community. By amplifying their voices, speakers advocate for enhanced healthcare services, improved access to treatment options, and increased availability of supportive care resources.

Several cancer support groups and advocacy organisations offer individuals chances to engage in public speaking. These platforms provide training, guidance, and support to speakers to ensure their stories are effectively conveyed and impactful. Public speaking plays a vital role in educational campaigns focused on increasing awareness about cancer prevention, early detection, and survivorship. Speakers contribute to community health initiatives and advocate for positive health behaviours.

Public speaking is a transformative form of community and social engagement for individuals affected by cancer. By sharing personal experiences, insights, and lessons learned, speakers inspire others, raise awareness, and build supportive networks within the cancer community. Public speaking empowers individuals to advocate for improved healthcare, challenge stigma, and promote a culture of compassion and understanding surrounding cancer.

95. Fundraising for Research: Contributing to Cancer Research Funding

Fundraising for cancer research is a vital form of community and social engagement that enables individuals and communities to actively contribute to advancing scientific knowledge, improving treatment options, and ultimately finding cures for cancer. By organising and participating in fundraising events, individuals not only raise financial support but also raise awareness, build solidarity within their communities, and inspire hope for a future free of cancer.

Cancer research fundraising initiatives generate funds that support pioneering research projects focused on uncovering the origins of cancer, pioneering new treatments, and enhancing patient outcomes. Each donation contributes directly to scientific progress and medical breakthroughs. Fundraising activities mobilise communities, uniting individuals, families, businesses, and organisations in a common goal to combat cancer. These events cultivate a sense of solidarity, purpose, and collective effort, empowering participants to create a significant difference in the battle against cancer.

Community-oriented events like charity walks, runs, cycling events, gala dinners, and bake sales are widely embraced for raising funds for cancer research. These initiatives not only secure donations but also serve as platforms for education, commemoration, and community bonding within the cancer community. Collaborations with businesses and corporations, achieved through sponsorship, employee-driven fundraising campaigns, and cause-related marketing efforts, further boost fundraising endeavours. Corporate partnerships elevate visibility, broaden outreach, and bolster financial support directed towards advancing cancer research.

Contributions to cancer research organisations and institutions play a pivotal role in funding essential laboratory investigations, clinical trials, and translational research endeavours. These donations expedite the advancement of novel therapies, diagnostic innovations, and preventive measures that yield global benefits for cancer patients. Certain fundraising campaigns also allocate resources to bolster support services for cancer patients and their families, encompassing vital provisions such as counselling, transportation aid, financial assistance, and survivorship initiatives. These comprehensive services significantly enhance quality of life and deliver holistic support across every phase of the cancer experience.

Fundraising events function as forums to raise awareness about cancer prevention, early detection, treatment choices, and survivorship. Participants and supporters transform into advocates for cancer awareness, promoting health screenings and healthy living habits among others. These events also celebrate collective accomplishments and milestones in the battle against cancer. They honour the commitment of volunteers, donors, researchers, healthcare providers, and advocates who play pivotal roles in advancing cancer research and enhancing patient outcomes.

Fundraising for cancer research is a powerful expression of community and social engagement, enabling individuals and communities to make a tangible impact in the fight against cancer. By organising and

96. Creating Art: Expressing Oneself Through Creative Arts

Creating art is a therapeutic and empowering form of community and social engagement for individuals affected by cancer. Whether through visual arts, music, writing, or performing arts, artistic expression provides a creative outlet for processing emotions, fostering self-discovery, and connecting with others. Art not only enhances psychological well-being but also promotes healing, resilience, and a sense of community among participants.

Therapeutic Benefits of Artistic Expression

Emotional Expression: Art allows individuals to explore and express complex emotions related to their cancer journey, including fear, hope, joy, and resilience. Through creative expression, individuals can articulate feelings that may be difficult to convey verbally, facilitating emotional catharsis and healing.

Stress Reduction: Engaging in artistic activities such as painting, drawing, sculpting, or playing musical instruments promotes relaxation and reduces stress levels. Artistic expression can serve as a form of mindfulness, helping individuals focus on the present moment and alleviate anxiety associated with cancer diagnosis and treatment.

Artistic workshops and classes designed for cancer patients, survivors, and caregivers offer a nurturing space for creative expression and skill enhancement. These sessions foster collaboration, peer encouragement, and shared learning among participants. Showcasing artwork and performances crafted by those affected by cancer not only celebrates artistic accomplishments but also raises awareness about the profound impact of cancer on individuals and communities. Exhibitions and performances serve as venues for storytelling, advocacy, and meaningful community conversations.

Art exhibitions, performances, and community projects centered on cancer themes play a vital role in educating the public about cancer prevention, early detection, treatment options, and survivorship. Artistic creations convey compelling messages, confront stereotypes, and drive positive societal shifts. Through artistic expression, individuals impacted by cancer reclaim their narratives and affirm their identities beyond the disease. These creative endeavours empower patients and survivors to champion their concerns, share personal stories, and provide inspiration to others navigating similar challenges.

Many healthcare institutions provide art therapy programs as integral components of their cancer care offerings. These programs are led by skilled therapists who assist participants in utilising art to delve into emotions, develop coping strategies, and enhance their quality of life throughout their treatment journey and beyond. Collaborations among healthcare providers, community groups, and artists facilitate interdisciplinary efforts to incorporate art into supportive care services. Such initiatives promote patient-centered approaches, support holistic well-being, and address the psychosocial challenges faced by individuals affected by cancer.

Creating art is a transformative form of community and social engagement for individuals affected by cancer, offering therapeutic benefits, fostering community connections, and raising awareness through creative expression. Artistic endeavours empower individuals to heal, advocate for change, and inspire hope in the face of adversity, demonstrating the profound impact of art in the fight against cancer.

97. Writing a Book: Documenting the Cancer Journey

Writing a book about one's cancer journey is a profound form of community and social engagement that not only documents personal experiences but also inspires, educates, and connects with others facing similar challenges. Whether it's a memoir, a collection of essays, or a practical guide, the act of writing provides individuals with cancer an opportunity to share their stories, insights, and lessons learned, fostering empathy and understanding within the broader community.

Writing serves as a profound tool for individuals to contemplate their cancer diagnosis, treatment journeys, and emotional paths. It offers a dedicated outlet to process intricate feelings, confront fears, and mark significant achievements, fostering personal development and resilience. Memoirs and books authored by cancer patients, survivors, caregivers, and healthcare providers serve as invaluable educational materials. They offer firsthand insights into navigating healthcare systems, making treatment choices, managing side effects, and coping with cancer's impact on everyday life.

Authoring a book presents avenues to connect with others impacted by cancer. Writers frequently discover solidarity and support from readers who relate to their stories, cultivating community and lessening feelings of loneliness. Cancer-themed books serve to educate about the disease's realities, dispel misunderstandings, and champion enhanced healthcare policies and support systems. Authors often evolve into advocates for cancer awareness, prevention, early detection, and patient-focused healthcare.

Impact on Others and the Community

Inspiration and Hope: Cancer survivors who share their stories inspire hope and offer reassurance to individuals currently undergoing treatment or facing uncertain outcomes. Readers find comfort in knowing they are not alone in their struggles and are inspired by stories of resilience and survival.

Education for Healthcare Providers: Books written by patients and caregivers provide healthcare professionals with insights into the lived experiences of those affected by cancer. This firsthand knowledge can inform compassionate and patient-centered care practices.

Writing as Therapy and Healing:

Catharsis: Writing offers therapeutic benefits by allowing authors to articulate their thoughts and emotions in a structured and meaningful way. It serves as a form of self-expression, emotional release, and healing during and after cancer treatment.

Legacy and Remembrance: For some individuals, writing a book serves as a legacy—a way to leave a lasting imprint and share wisdom with future generations. It honours the journey of resilience and courage in navigating life with cancer.

Sharing personal experiences in a book demands courage and vulnerability. Authors may confront fears of judgment or reliving painful memories, yet often draw strength from reader support and the therapeutic act of writing itself. Completing and publishing a book stands as a notable accomplishment, marking personal milestones and honouring the bravery and resilience needed to confront the trials of cancer.

Writing a book about the cancer journey is a powerful form of community and social engagement that empowers individuals to share their stories, educate others, build connections, and advocate for change. Through storytelling, authors offer insights, hope, and support to fellow patients, survivors, caregivers, and healthcare professionals, contributing to a more compassionate and informed understanding of cancer in society.

98. Starting a Blog: Sharing the Journey Online

Starting a blog about your cancer journey is a dynamic and impactful way to engage with the community, share experiences, provide support, and raise awareness. In the digital age, blogging offers a platform for individuals affected by cancer to connect with a global audience, document their experiences in real-time, and contribute to a supportive online community.

Creating a Supportive Community:

Connecting with Others: A cancer blog serves as a virtual support network where individuals can connect with fellow patients, survivors, caregivers, and advocates worldwide. It fosters a sense of belonging and understanding among those navigating similar challenges.

Sharing Experiences: Blogging allows individuals to share their personal stories, challenges, triumphs, and insights. By documenting their journey in detail, bloggers offer a candid and authentic portrayal of life with cancer, breaking down stigma and providing valuable perspective to readers.

Education and Awareness:

Informing Others: Cancer blogs educate readers about the realities of the disease, treatment options, side effects, and lifestyle adjustments. They provide firsthand accounts of medical appointments, procedures, and emotional experiences, offering practical information and emotional support to individuals at different stages of their cancer journey.

Advocacy: Bloggers often become advocates for cancer awareness, early detection, patient rights, and healthcare reform. They use their platform to raise awareness about important issues, share resources, and promote initiatives that benefit the cancer community.

Blogging empowers individuals by providing a voice and platform to share their thoughts, emotions, and perspectives on navigating life with cancer. It serves as a tool for self-expression, emotional processing, and personal development throughout the cancer journey. Regularly writing blog posts promotes self-reflection and introspection, enabling bloggers to document progress, mark milestones, and delve into the emotional and psychological dimensions of their experience, thereby enhancing resilience and emotional well-being.

Blogging fosters interaction and engagement with readers through comments, emails, and social media, cultivating meaningful relationships and a supportive online community. It encourages connections where individuals offer encouragement, advice, and solidarity. Blogs also facilitate communication between patients and healthcare providers, allowing bloggers to share treatment insights, provide feedback on healthcare services, and advocate for patient-centered care practices.

Bloggers face the delicate task of balancing transparency with privacy, sharing personal experiences while respecting boundaries. They often opt to anonymise specific details or emphasise particular aspects of their journey to safeguard their privacy and that of their loved ones. A cancer blog can create a lasting impact by documenting one's journey, insights, and contributions to the cancer community. It serves as a legacy of courage, resilience, and advocacy for future readers and those touched by cancer.

Starting a blog about your cancer journey is a powerful form of community and social engagement that empowers individuals to share their experiences, educate others, build connections, and advocate for change. Through blogging, individuals affected by cancer create a supportive and informative online presence, offering encouragement, resources, and solidarity to fellow patients, survivors, caregivers, and healthcare professionals worldwide.

Miscellaneous

99. Using Alternative Therapies with Caution: Always Consulting with Healthcare Professionals

When facing cancer, individuals often explore alternative therapies alongside conventional treatments to improve their quality of life, manage symptoms, and support overall well-being. While alternative therapies can offer complementary benefits, it's crucial to approach them with caution and always consult healthcare professionals to ensure safety and compatibility with ongoing treatments.

Alternative therapies, including acupuncture, herbal supplements, and mindfulness practices, complement conventional medical treatments to provide holistic care for cancer patients. These therapies can alleviate treatment side effects, reduce stress, and enhance emotional well-being. The spectrum of alternative therapies encompasses various practices such as acupuncture, massage therapy, dietary supplements, meditation, yoga, and energy healing, each targeting different dimensions of physical, emotional, and spiritual health.

Healthcare professionals are essential in incorporating alternative therapies into comprehensive cancer treatment strategies. They offer expertise, personalised guidance, and recommendations tailored to individual health conditions, treatment objectives, and potential interactions with conventional therapies. Collaborating with oncologists, integrative medicine specialists, and other healthcare providers ensures that alternative therapies are safe, evidence-based, and consistent with established treatment protocols. Healthcare professionals also monitor treatment effectiveness, address potential side effects, and adapt therapies as necessary to maximise patient outcomes.

Potential Benefits and Considerations:

Symptom Management: Alternative therapies may alleviate cancer-related symptoms such as pain, fatigue, nausea, and anxiety. For example, acupuncture and massage therapy can promote relaxation, reduce pain perception, and improve overall quality of life during treatment.

Emotional Support: Mindfulness practices, meditation, and support groups offer emotional support and help patients cope with the psychological impact of cancer diagnosis and treatment. These therapies promote resilience, emotional well-being, and a positive outlook on recovery.

Critical Evaluation:

While certain alternative therapies have shown positive outcomes in clinical trials, others may lack strong scientific backing for their effectiveness or safety. Therefore, it's crucial for patients and healthcare providers to carefully assess available research, peer-reviewed studies, and reliable sources of information before integrating alternative therapies into treatment regimens. Approaches like herbal supplements and dietary interventions have the potential to interact with prescribed medications, impact treatment effectiveness, or worsen underlying health issues. Healthcare professionals diligently monitor for possible drug interactions and adverse effects, ensuring informed decision-making and personalised treatment plans.

Informed Decision-Making: Patients are encouraged to actively participate in treatment decisions, discuss goals and preferences with healthcare providers, and seek reliable information from reputable sources. Open communication fosters mutual respect, trust, and collaborative care between patients and healthcare teams.

Holistic Approach: Integrating alternative therapies within a holistic cancer care framework acknowledges the interconnectedness of physical, emotional, and spiritual dimensions of health. This patient-centered approach promotes personalised care, enhances treatment adherence, and supports overall well-being throughout the cancer journey.

Using alternative therapies with caution involves informed decision-making, collaborative communication with healthcare professionals, and a commitment to safety, efficacy, and patient-centered care. By integrating evidence-based alternative therapies alongside conventional treatments, individuals affected by cancer can enhance their quality of life, manage symptoms, and support overall health and well-being in a comprehensive and balanced manner.

100. Sodium Bicarbonate and Cancer Treatment

While Bicarbonate of soda is great for fungal infections like smelly feet and armpits, some proponents suggest that sodium bicarbonate can increase the pH of tumours, making the environment less favourable for cancer cells to thrive.

This theory is based on the idea that cancer cells prefer an acidic environment.

Scientific Evidence

Preclinical Studies: Some laboratory studies have shown that alkalising agents like sodium bicarbonate can slow the growth of certain cancer cells in petri dishes or animal models. However, these studies are not conclusive and do not necessarily translate to effectiveness in humans.

Clinical Trials: There is a lack of robust clinical evidence supporting the use of sodium bicarbonate in treating cancer in humans. No large-scale, peer-reviewed clinical trials have demonstrated that sodium bicarbonate is effective or safe for cancer treatment.

Potential Risks:

Alkalosis: Excessive consumption of sodium bicarbonate can lead to metabolic alkalosis, a condition where the body's pH becomes too high. This can cause symptoms like muscle twitching, hand tremors, light-headedness, nausea, and can be potentially life-threatening.

Electrolyte Imbalance: High doses of sodium bicarbonate can disrupt the balance of electrolytes in the body, leading to issues such as low potassium levels (hypokalaemia), which can cause heart problems.

Interactions with Other Treatments: Sodium bicarbonate may interact with other cancer treatments, potentially reducing their effectiveness or increasing toxicity.

Medical Guidance

It is crucial to rely on treatments that are supported by scientific evidence and prescribed by healthcare professionals. Conventional cancer treatments, such as surgery, radiation therapy, chemotherapy, immunotherapy, and targeted therapy, have been extensively researched and have demonstrated effectiveness and safety profiles.

While sodium bicarbonate has some antifungal properties, its use in treating cancer is not supported by scientific evidence and can be potentially harmful. It's essential to consult with a healthcare professional before considering any alternative treatments, especially for serious conditions like cancer.

101. Staying Informed: Keeping Up to Date with the Latest Research and Treatment Options

In the realm of cancer treatment and management, staying informed about the latest research and treatment options is crucial for patients, caregivers, and healthcare professionals alike. This proactive approach empowers individuals affected by cancer to make informed decisions, explore innovative therapies, and advocate for personalised care that aligns with their unique health needs and treatment goals.

Importance of Staying Informed

Access to Cutting-Edge Therapies: Advances in medical research continually introduce new diagnostic tools, treatment modalities, and therapeutic approaches for various types of cancer. Staying informed enables patients and healthcare providers to explore cutting-edge therapies that may offer improved outcomes, reduced side effects, and enhanced quality of life.

Evidence-Based Decision Making: Accessing up-to-date information on clinical trials, treatment guidelines, and scientific discoveries allows patients to make evidence-based decisions in collaboration with their healthcare team. This informed approach supports treatment adherence, personalised care planning, and proactive management of cancer-related challenges.

Participating in clinical trials provides access to novel treatments and experimental therapies that may not be widely available. Staying informed about ongoing trials, eligibility criteria, and potential benefits allows patients to consider innovative treatment options under the guidance of healthcare professionals.

Second Opinions: Seeking second opinions from specialised oncologists and multidisciplinary teams helps patients explore diverse perspectives on diagnosis, treatment plans, and therapeutic alternatives. Staying informed facilitates comprehensive evaluations of treatment options and fosters informed decision-making based on expert insights.

Accessing reliable sources such as medical journals, peer-reviewed articles, and patient advocacy groups empowers individuals to broaden their understanding of medical topics and assert their health rights. By fostering open communication with healthcare providers, patients can participate in shared decision-making, cultivate mutual respect, and engage in collaborative care. Keeping informed allows individuals to actively contribute to treatment conversations, express preferences, and shape personalised care plans that align with their values and treatment goals.

Remaining knowledgeable about supportive care options, survivorship programs, and integrative therapies improves the overall quality of life during the cancer experience. Access to comprehensive support systems that cater to physical, emotional, and psychosocial needs fosters holistic well-being and strengthens resilience. Informed individuals affected by cancer can advocate for enhanced healthcare policies, affordable treatment options, and community support programs. Promoting awareness about cancer prevention, early detection, and advancements in treatment enhances public education and empowers communities.

Embracing a proactive approach to staying informed involves continuous learning, adaptation to evolving treatment standards, and proactive engagement with healthcare advancements. Patients and caregivers navigate the complexities of cancer care with resilience, optimism, and a commitment to informed decision-making.

Staying informed about the latest research and treatment options empowers individuals affected by cancer to actively participate in their care journey, explore innovative therapies, and advocate for personalised treatment approaches. By embracing a proactive stance, staying connected with healthcare professionals, and accessing reliable information sources, patients and caregivers navigate the complexities of cancer treatment with confidence, resilience, and hope for improved outcomes and quality of life.

Conclusion

As we conclude this journey through 101 different ways to fight cancer, remember that each person's path is unique. The strategies, tips, and insights shared here are meant to inspire and empower you on your own journey toward healing and resilience.

Cancer may be a formidable opponent, but through knowledge, determination, and the support of loved ones and healthcare professionals, it can be faced with courage. Each day is an opportunity to incorporate new practices, embrace hope, and cherish moments of joy.

Above all, remember that you are not alone. Millions around the world are navigating similar paths, and together, we continue to push boundaries, advocate for better treatments, and work towards a future where cancer is not feared but understood and overcome.

May this book serve as a beacon of hope and a guidepost in your fight against cancer. Your journey is a testament to strength, resilience, and the power of community. Keep fighting, keep believing, and keep living each day to the fullest.